D1708451

WITHDRAWN

Aging Parents, Ambivalent Baby Boomers:
A CRITICAL APPROACH TO GERONTOLOGY

THE REYNOLDS SERIES IN SOCIOLOGY
Larry T. Reynolds, *Editor*
by **GENERAL HALL, INC.**

AGING PARENTS, AMBIVALENT BABY BOOMERS:

A CRITICAL APPROACH TO GERONTOLOGY

Jayne E. Maugans
Houghton College

GENERAL HALL, INC.
Publishers
5 Talon Way
Dix Hills, New York 11746

AGING PARENTS, AMBIVALENT BABY BOOMERS:
A Critical Approach To Gerontology

GENERAL HALL, INC.
5 Talon Way
Dix Hills, New York 11746

Copyright © 1994 by General Hall, Inc.

All rights reserved. No part of this publication may be
reproduced, stored in a retrieval system or transmitted
in any form or by any means, except for the inclusion of
brief quotations in a review, without the prior permission
of the publisher.

Publisher: Ravi Mehra
Editor: Kristen Kelley
Composition: Graphics Division, General Hall, Inc.

LIBRARY OF CONGRESS CATALOG CARD NUMBER: 93–79472

ISBN: 0–930390–23–7 [paper]
       0–930390–49–0 [cloth]

HQ
1063.6
.M38
1994

Manufactured in the United States of America

For Elena Bastida

Contents

ACKNOWLEDGMENTS

The idea for this book did not just come to me; it was a process shaped by the collective exchanges I had with many persons for several years. It began when I was working on my master's degree at Wichita State University, studying under Dr. Elena Bastida and Dr. Robert Allegrucci. These two individuals prepared me for further study in critical theory and aging, opening my mind and sociological eye to human suffering and the possibilities for social change.

After completing my master's degree, my education was advanced at the State University of New York at Buffalo under Dr. Ben Agger. He is the most influential person behind this work. I am particularly grateful to Ben for his support and intervention throughout the writing of this book. He helped me, first, by guiding me through the critical theory literature, and second, by bringing the proposed manuscript to the attention of the publisher and, finally, reviewing an early draft of the work. His recommendations were most useful to me.

A word of special appreciation is also extended to Dr. Beth Anne Shelton for her many cogent criticisms from the proposal to a later draft. Others from Buffalo, New York, who deserve mention include Judge Barbara Howe and Dr. Lionel Lewis. All these individuals offered their time and assistance to help me clarify my position in the book, and for this I am thankful.

The most insightful review of the initial manuscript came from Dr. Raymond Morrow. I am indebted to him for his copious comments and suggestions, which I found to be legitimate, enlightening, and worthy of pursuit.

Three individuals who were instrumental in the editing of this book are Larry Reynolds, Sharon Hoover, and Irene Glynn. Their conscientious remarks tremendously improved the reading of the book.

Two people in the Social Science Department at Alfred University deserve recognition for their assistance. Dr. Steve Peterson arranged for me to use the Alfred facilities and staff in completing the final mailing of the book to the publisher. In this endeavor, Karen Mix was most giving.

I also want to thank the fifty baby boomers who participated, without reward, in the research (at the time of the study, I was a doctoral student without funding to pass on to my participants). I hope in completing the research, I have given something back to each and every one of them.

Finally, I wish to thank my husband, Bob Scherzer, for his patience and relentless support throughout the writing of this book. And, of course, a word of praise to my parents, Clyde and Shirley Maugans, for always making me feel I could accomplish a major undertaking if I wanted to.

INTRODUCTION

Something is happening in America: There are more adult children with living parents than ever before. This adult child population, commonly referred to as the "baby boom generation," has had unprecedented life experiences. From birth these children have been the center of attention of one institution after another—hospitals, schools, the law, and always Madison Avenue.

According to Jones (1980), the baby boom in the United States began in 1946 when births soared to an all-time high of 3.4 million, peaked in 1957 when 4.3 million babies were born, and ended in 1964. By 1970, there were some 20 million teenagers in this country, and more to come. In terms of population pyramids, the baby boom cohort is characterized as a "pig going through a python." Actually, demographers frequently divide the baby boom into two waves: the first from 1946 to 1957 and the second from 1958 to 1964. This book is concerned with the first wave, now composed of women and men well into adulthood.

Beyond its size, the baby boom generation is historically unique because it was the first American generation to be raised in a postindustrial society with accelerating changes: the first generation to go from the crib to college watching television; the last generation to be reared by housewives; the generation that took to the streets in the 1960s and 1970s to protest the Vietnam war and to support the rights of women, blacks, Latinos, Native Americans, gays, animals, forests, and whales; the first generation to have as part of its culture a counterculture embracing peace, love, and "let it be," while rejecting such sacred societal institutions as the military and marriage; the first generation to be twice as likely to go to college as its parents, and to find that higher education does not necessarily lead to career opportunities and advancements (Jones 1980).

Compared to other generations, the baby boom generation has the highest rates for postponing marriage, having dual-career marriages, preventing pregnancy, getting divorced, heading single-

1

parent households, being depressed, and committing suicide (Jones 1980). As a whole, the generation has valued and still values youth and self-expression. It is a generation that entered adulthood during the "me decade," asking, "What's in it for me?" It is a generation concerned with personal fulfillment—in their sex lives, finances, health, and interpersonal relations.

Now, as baby boomers near or nestle into midlife, there are concerns about relationships with aging parents: Did the turbulence of the teenage years irrevocably sever the bonds between them and their parents? Are they too busy with child rearing and careers to take time out for moms and dads? Are their personal lives in such turmoil that they do not have the time or energy to devote to relationships with their parents? Have they moved so far away that they cannot be a part of their parents' lives? Have differences in values distanced the older and younger generations? Have the baby boomers come to regard institutionalized care of the aged as more desirable than other options? Are they too concerned with themselves to care about the people who raised them? Are they simply not interested in their parents?

Even before baby boomers reached adulthood, there was a growing awareness of the "aging of America" and with it an interest in relations between adult children and their aging parents. Publications, ranging from self-help manuals to scholarly works, presented a loud and clear message: The adult child/parent relationship in the United States is strained by rapid changes within the society, by "modernization." Typically, sociologists and psychologists conducting intergenerational studies concerned with how well adult children have overcome the social and psychological obstacles of modern life assume that modern life is detrimental to a healthy adult child/parent relationship.

The prevailing theme resonating throughout mainstream literature on intergenerational relations is that the successful adaptation of adult children to modern life is crucial for good intergenerational relationships. Although difficulties encountered by adult children in their parental relationships are approached as consequences of modern America, overcoming them is regarded as the younger generation's responsibility. Concern is with identifying strains, the trends leading to them, and possible solutions for overcoming adaptation problems.

Filial adaptation is the term I have coined to refer to the ongoing adjustments adult children are expected to make to their contemporary environments in order to have close and caring relationships with their parents (relationships based on sentiments of love and attachment and a willingness to provide support and aid to parents). It includes adult children responding to unprecedented demographic, economic, and cultural changes, such as the well-known "aging of America," the familiar fiscal crisis, and the infamous "me mentality."

That Americans are interested in filial adaptation is clear, judging by the numerous newspaper and magazine articles written for adult children about aging parents. In popular journalism, the intent is to bridge the generation gap by enlightening the younger generation to facts on aging in America. Book stores display such titles as *Aging Parents, Our Aging Parents, Helping Elderly Parents, Caring for Your Aged Parents, Understanding Your Aging Parents,* and *When Your Parents Grow Old.*

Problems of Mainstream Social Gerontology

In responding to the growing public interest in the adult child/parent relationship, social gerontologists have attempted to explain how the relationship is faring in modern society, how it has changed since the dawning of the industrial revolution, and what dynamics it will likely take in the future. Nonetheless, they have typically confined the character of the intergenerational relationship, past, present, and future, to the realm of quantification—for example, demographics on older parents, sibling, and women in the work force; counts of phone calls, letters, and visits exchanged between generations; and measures of miles between the two households.

In studying filial adaptation, researchers in social gerontology emphasize the individual as the unit of analysis and adaptation as the key to successful intergenerational relations. Researchers analyze adult children's social roles and responsibilities, resources, and personal development, then correlate the extent to which they have close and caring relationships with their parents. But, the analyses ignore the fact that the social organization of the modern society under study is capitalist patriarchy.

Thus, modern society (and its various social arrangements) is presented as a social fact, an inevitable social reality. The sociohistorical and the sociopolitical compositions of the society are not at issue, all that matters is that the society is "modern." This steers the problem away from the political arena and into that of the personal. As a result, disharmony between generations can and is addressed as a private rather than a public problem because the problem becomes, not the modern society that is inevitable, but adult children, for they alone can change, accommodate, adapt.

By mapping filial adaptation alongside modernity, the problem becomes one of "role strain," "limited resources," or "immaturity" in so-called contemporary society, industrial society, or advanced society. The solution to the problem, therefore, is to help adult children help themselves adapt to the given society without a radical transformation of either the individual or the society. Not surprisingly, the usual summaries in mainstream publications are limited to either self-help solutions that solidify the current social structure or to policy recommendations that call for innocuous changes in the social system (e.g., more funding for senior service programs).

Political economists of aging, theorists outside the mainstream whose analysis includes a study of the "interrelationships between the polity, economy, and society, or more specifically, the reciprocal influences among government . . . the economy, social classes, state, and status groups," point out that the dominant theoretical approaches to the study of aging stress "adjustment" as the nexus of successful aging experiences (Minkler 1984, 11). Their search for the causes behind the problems of aging, which includes intergenerational conflict, has led political economists to a critique of the capitalist system's manner of prioritizing and allocating scarce resources, especially as reflected in federal budgets of advanced industrialized nations (Minkler 1984; Estes & Newcomer 1983; Myles 1984).

The mainstream approach has been, nonetheless, effective in describing aspects of aging of America, including demographic trends, statistics surrounding the institutionalization, health, employment, retirement, and long-term care of the aged in the United States. Leading works have identified many myths about aging, stereotypes of the elderly, and troubles of the aged and their caretakers, making a major contribution to social gerontology that has directly affected, for the better, the quality of life of many older Americans and their families.

While much has been offered in the principal literature about the problem of filial adaptation in terms of demographics and individual deficits, little has been added to our knowledge about filial adaptation as an object located in a particular social organization. In every theoretical framework outlined by traditional social gerontologists—structural functionalism, symbolic interactionism, exchange theory, or life-cycle—modern society is regarded as a given, and therefore our understanding of intergenerational relations in the United States is biased in the sense that it is slanted toward an assumed relationship within an advanced capitalist patriarchal society.

I believe that because social gerontologists have ignored the particular social organization of their subject, namely, advanced capitalist patriarchy, they have proceeded with very definite assumptions about the nature of intergenerational relations, even though they have yet to state their underlying assumptions. The purpose of this work is to articulate these assumptions, to explore their theoretical foundations (for, as Adorno wrote, "what a theory regards and disregards determines its quality"), and to present a comparative analysis of the adult child/parent relationship using a sample from the baby boom generation.

As I see it, the two predominant assumptions behind the traditional notion of filial adaptation are that (1) the adult child should adapt to modern American life, rather than the other way around; and (2) the adult child/parent relationship should be a nearly perfect relationship within society as it now exists. In both cases, modern American society is presented as a social fact, an inevitable social reality; therefore, responsibility for harmonious intergenerational relations is placed on the adult child, who must adapt to the status quo without any expectation of a significant transformation of the larger social organization of society. In both situations, the adult child (not society) is expected to adapt, to be nearly perfect. In short, filial adaptation, as approached by the traditionalists, is not a political subject.

Ideological versus Critical Theory

I am suggesting that the above assumptions stem from theories that are ideological rather than critical. Borrowing Osmond's (1987) definition, ideological theories are theories that "present the social structure ahistorically, as a natural, inevitable, unchangeable or universal feature of human existence . . . (and) legitimize and reinforce the given system, regardless of that system's deficiencies." Ideological theories also repress "the possibility of historical alternatives"; they "simultaneously provide an interpretation of the present and offer, through this interpretation, the future as the extrapolation of an existing trend" (Osmond 1987; Poster 1978). Ideological theories disregard the sociohistorical context of their subject matter, legitimize the existing social order, and quell alternative explanations and possibilities for tomorrow. I view the ongoing theoretical orientations in social gerontology as ideological because they approach filial adaptation as if it were a necessary phenomenon. In doing so, they justify existing social relations in the United States and blind their proponents and others to a variety of options.

In contrast, there are theories that do not allow for a society or any of its aspects to be accepted as a given. These theories, known as critical theories, call for a comprehensive understanding of social life that requires theorists to derive their explanations of the social world from a historical analysis encompassing the whole organization of human existence (Horkheimer 1972). Critical theorists probe beyond the quantitative to identifying that which qualifies the underlying relations between people, the subjective, emotional, and psychological, considered within the total historical sphere of a society. Such probing helps uncover the realities of human relations, especially forces of domination and potential forces of freedom.

Critical theories also differ from ideological theories in that they regard private disorders as reflecting general disorders and thus see them as political disorders (Marcuse 1955; Jacoby 1975). For critical theorists, ascribing the problems of life to the individual without reference to the society justifies and advances a retarded state of society. Hence, the whole notion of filial adaptation is suspect for those who do not accept as given the current social organization of society and who regard the private as a reflection of the public.

Critical theories allow us to challenge the assumptions about the nature of intergenerational relations underlying mainstream social gerontology. The key to this challenge lies in looking at the emotional character of the adult child/parent relationship and seeing if it is perhaps not simply a product of modernization but of a specific social organization: capitalist patriarchy. Another way is to refute the proposition that modernization alone has undermined the adult child/parent relationship in the United States, and one way of doing this is by testing some of the modernization factors frequently cited as salient for the demise of intergenerational harmony.

My objective is to challenge assumptions about filial adaptation underlying mainstream social gerontology. I intend to reveal the narrow scope of the established gerontological orientation and then go beyond it by analyzing the relationship among baby boomers and their parents within the context of capitalist patriarchy. In other words, I seek to understand filial adaptation from a critical, rather than a traditional perspective, which I believe will bring a fresh approach to the study of intergenerational relations in social gerontology.

Explaining filial adaptation is a theoretical problem of major significance for sociology and its subfield, social gerontology. As a discipline, sociology is concerned with the study of human arrangements and, ultimately, their affects on the individual. In traditional sociology, concern is with addressing individual problems without disrupting the established social order. In the same tradition, typical works in mainstream social gerontology approach filial adaptation as an individual problem that can be minimized by minor adjustments to the system. In contrast, critical theory regards personal problems as political problems. Hence, the critical approach is concerned with radical change not only in the individual but in the social order as well.

Part I of this book includes the critical theoretical approach to the study of family relations and the qualitative data from interviews I had with fifty baby boomers during 1989. Specifics of the sample are presented in Chapter 10.

In Chapter 1, a critical theoretical view of human nature is discussed. The chapter reviews the heritage and the legacy of the critical approach to the study of family relations, beginning with the ideas of Karl Marx and Friedrich Engels, continuing with the Frankfurt School, Mark Poster, and Christopher Lasch, and ending with feminist critical thought.

Chapter 2 explores ways in which to diminish the ambivalence of adult children. Criticized is the hierarchical, authoritarian structure of the present-day family under capitalist patriarchy. The importance of changing the social demands on the individual is stressed, emphasizing how the personal is political. Excerpts from the baby boomers reveal ways in which the intergenerational relationship can be less exploitative.

In Chapters 3 through 7, responses surrounding the strain in the intergenerational relationship are presented and analyzed. Underscored is the oppressive arrangement in the family and other human relations in American society, particularly those surrounding authority and sexual differentials. The ambivalence of baby boomers is revealed and explained in the context of the social demands placed on them under capitalist patriarchy. Chapter 7 ends with possibilities for overcoming oppressive social relations.

Part II covers the mainstream explanations of intergenerational relations in the United States. Chapter 8 reviews the current research in mainstream social gerontology on the adult child/parent relationship. In Chapter 9, the explanations of intergenerational relations as based in ideological theory are reviewed, and ideological theory of the family from its beginning to the present is identified. The quantitative findings from the interviews with the baby boomers are presented in Chapter 10, offered in challenge of the mainstream approach.

PART I

BABY BOOMERS' AMBIVALENCE: QUALITATIVE FINDINGS

1 CRITICAL THOUGHT ON
INTERGENERATIONAL
RELATIONS

Without question, there have been dramatic changes in American society over the past century, particularly in terms of its size, technological advances, work force composition, state policies, and monopolistic practices. These changes have had a direct impact on the American family, but I find the mainstream's explanations of them in regard to the adult child/parent relationship dimsighted, mainly because these accounts approach the changes as "social facts" without "social origins." In the established academy of social gerontology, family life and society are described as if each were a natural and predictable phenomenon and the relation between them fixed. Left in a haze is the history behind the larger forces affecting the makeup of society and their ultimate impact on intergenerational relations and without the history, solutions are spiritless. The problem lies with theoretical frameworks that do not discern between natural forces and created ones, between a fact of life and a fact of establishment.

Critical theorists, in contrast, see the nature of the difference, and they write about it both in critiques of traditional theories that deny the historically constructed component of human relations and in explanation of their own dialectical method. Max Horkheimer's lengthy explanation of "human nature" is a good example of the critical theorists' reasoning on this point:

> The term "human nature" here does not refer to an original or an eternal or a uniform essence. Every philosophical doctrine which sees the movement of society or the life of the individual as emerging out of a fundamental, historical unity is open to justified criticism. Such theories with their undialectical method have special difficulty in coming to gripswith the fact that new individual and social qualities arise in the

10

historical process. Their reaction to this fact either takes the form of mechanical evolution: all human characteristics which arise at a later point were originally present in germ; or it takes the form of some variety of philosophical anthropology: these characteristics emerge from a metaphysical "ground" of being. (1980,118)

The alternative view of human nature is a continuation of arguments presented in the nineteenth century by Karl Marx. In the *Grundrisse*, Marx blasted political economists of the time for presenting the individual as being "in conformity with nature" and as confronting "forms of social union . . . as an external necessity," thereby creating the illusion that human nature is without history. The obvious to Marx is that human relations would not exist if the individual were in isolation; it is because of the unique social organization of society that the individual and, moreover, social relations develop. Human nature is not a fact of nature but of history.

Marx's subjectivist message is this: Because social relations are social products, they can be reproduced in such a way that all instead of a few benefit from them; the key to emancipation lies in people becoming conscious of this fact and acting accordingly. As Marx saw it, capitalist society stultifies and objectifies the essential nature of humans, creating a condition in which people become estranged from their work and social existence; he called this *alienation*. In the 1920s, Marx's message was expanded by Georg Lukacs's concepts reification and totality in *History and Class Consciousness* by Antonio Gramsci's ideological hegemony and praxis in *Selections from the Prison Notebooks*. These novel concepts are major contributions to critical notions about the meaning of nature.

The first concept, reification, refers to how humans have come to regard their activities and products as "things" separate from themselves, even though they have created them. What has happened, according to Lukacs, is that in the separation of producers from their products "all the social and economic conditions necessary for the emergence of modern capitalism tend to replace 'natural' relations which exhibit human relations more plainly by rationally reified relations" (1968, 91). In Lukacs's critique, traditional ideas about the nature of social reality are nothing more than mental semblances of the established; more succinctly, they are reified constructs.

The second concept, totality, meant to Lukacs, "the all-pervasive supremacy of the whole over the parts" (1968,27). According to Lukacs, a social phenomenon could not be studied as a single entity but must be considered in relation to the historical whole; otherwise, the structures of human civilization are perceived as things grown organically, not created by humans. Lukacs concluded that if a subject were studied in its totality, then the concept "nature" would take on this new meaning, which would help all of us out of our reified existence:

> Authentic humanity, the true essence of man liberated from the false, mechanising forms of society: man as a perfected whole who has inwardly overcome, or is in the process of overcoming, the dichotomies of theory and practice, reason and the senses, form and content; man whose tendency to create his own forms does not imply an abstract rationalism which ignores concrete content; man for whom freedom and necessity are identical. (1968, 136–37)

Gramsci likewise demonstrated the difference between a natural order and a created one. His argument includes viewing humans as entering relationships with one another, not nature, through their work and other activities. Human nature, as Gramsci wrote, "is not to be found in any one particular man but in the whole history of mankind" (1972, 80). It was important to Gramsci that the totality of social relations include not only how the relations exist but their genesis as well, because every individual is "not only the synthesis of existing relations but also the history of these relations" (1972, 78). In sum, human nature was to Gramsci historical development.

Gramsci took his views on nature and transposed them into an explanation of how power is legitimized in capitalist society. Accordingly, the ideas of the ruling class are always the ruling ideas of the time, a situation created and perpetuated by the ruling class through a belief system stressing the necessity for formal authority and discipline and resulting in the current order being perceived by all members of society as the correct and natural one, what Gramsci designated as ideological hegemony (Agger 1979; Osmond 1987; Ritzer 1983). As Gramsci saw it, the domination of one class over another in capitalist society is legitimized by ideological hegemony;

defying ideological hegemony would require praxis, that is, the interplay of theory and practice or the union of emancipatory ideas with emancipatory social action (Osmond 1987).

A few decades after Gramsci, Herbert Marcuse continued the critical crusade with an attack on the conventional works of his time. In *Negations* (1968), Marcuse claimed that in mainstream work, nature becomes a myth that hides the historical and social processes of human relations. In a later work, *Counterrevolution and Revolt* (1972), Marcuse would present nature as nothing more than an historical product, "subjected to a specific rationality which became, to an ever increasing extent, technological, instrumentalist rationality, bent to the requirements of capitalism." Marcuse then countered convention by establishing this relation between nature and freedom: Because nature is a historical entity, it can be transformed by humans into that which fosters freedom and happiness for all members of the society. The nature distinction survives today in Russell Jacoby's writings. In *Social Amnesia*, Jacoby defines nature as that which truly belongs to the "archaic and biological," in contrast to second nature, which refers to "history that has hardened into nature" (1975). In Jacoby's opinion, researchers who do not make the distinction between nature and second nature run the risk of presenting a social or psychological find as a natural find instead of what it is, a fossilized find; without an account of the historical organization of society, the end result is a static portrayal of human life that, for millions of people, is reified as reality.

With an understanding of the conceptual difference between nature and second nature, critical theorists have developed their own ideas about family relations. Unlike traditional theorists, critical theorists explore the relation between the individual and society, and through this exploration, come to test the posited natural existence of the family. One of their major premises is that all subject matter, including the family, must be viewed in its social totality, that is, taking into account its historically specific social formation, which includes all its facets: biological, cultural, historical, and otherwise. From another angle, it means that their subject cannot be comprehended if approached as an isolated phenomenon hence the antipositivist position of the critical theorists (Osmond 1987).

The theoretical goal of critical theorists is to construct a body of explanation of the social world that is sincere and truthful, one that will help make sense of the human condition and open the way for

reform that means real efforts to change society rather than superficial attempts to make people's behavior better. Since the goal is to
expose how the seemingly "natural" or "universal" are socially
produced, critical theorists study the social relation of interest in its
contemporary form, showing how it is related to the historical
whole.

To this end, critical theorists develop methods that they hope
will lead to a recapitulation of social relations stripped of synthetics,
presented on paper and in person as one, but only one insight into
reality. Their preferred technique, dialectics, tests the logic of the so-
called commonplace by revealing the opposite of the current social
relation (thus, the actual social relation). Dialectical thought, wrote
Marcuse, "starts with the experience that the world is unfree; that is
to say, man and nature exist in conditions of alienation . . ." The
power of dialectical thought lies in analyzing social relations in
terms of their internal inadequacies; this is effective in explaining
how the social relation is reproduced and how it has the potential to
change because of its internal contradictions (Osmond 1987). The
total contribution made in the area of family relations by critical
theorists is extensive. My review, however, is merely a rundown of
the essential ideas covered by critical thinkers beginning with Marx
and Engels, Lukacs, and Gramsci. Then the Frankfurt School is
discussed along with two authors, Poster and Lasch, and I end with
the work of feminist theorists.

The Beginnings of Critical Theory of the Family

As the historians Laslett & Wall (1972) explain, Karl Marx and
Friedrich Engels, unlike most of their contemporaries, did not
approach the monogamous family of contemporary Western Europe
as the family's highest evolutionary stage. Instead, they argued that
the familiar family form emerged simultaneously with private
property, the two being aspects of a specific stage in human
organization: capitalism. As Marx and Engels saw it, the family, as
it has become known, depends on productive relations; therefore,
universally speaking, the family could not have been fundamental to
society in all the various stages of human evolution.

In *Origin of the Family, Private Property and the State* (1884) the ideas of Marx and Engels were united by Engels into what has become the landmark work of critical theory on the family. Their thesis in a nutshell is that with the development of capitalism, the state rises, and as it does, the importance of "familism" relative to other institutions is reduced. Moreover, the family becomes a miniature model of the larger system of exploitative social relations; much is being said here that is worth further discussion.

First, the critical thesis claims that the state is a product of capitalism, which means it exists because of a type of economic development, not because of society itself. The position of Marx and Engels is that the state has not always existed, in fact, it did not exist in many societies, but it became necessary "with the cleavage of society into classes." Although the state appears "natural" to most citizens, it is a historical artifact created to keep in check class antagonism; the following quote, which must be read in its entirety, clarifies this point:

> The state is . . . a product of society at a certain stage of development; it is the admission that this society has become entangled in an insoluble contradiction with itself, that it is cleft into irreconcilable antagonisms which it is powerless to dispel. But in order that these antagonisms, classes with   conflicting economic interests, might not consume themselves and society in sterile struggle, a power seemingly standing above society became necessary for the purpose of moderating the conflict, of keeping it within the bounds of "order"; and this power, arisen out of society, but placing itself above it, and increasingly alienating itself from it, is the state. (1972,652)

Hence, from Marx and Engels's viewpoint, the state is superimposed on society; it is not a separate entity but one totally bound to the constructed inequalities inherent under capitalism. They believed that if class differentials were destroyed, the state would eventually disappear. To this task they looked to the proletariat, the working class of the world.

Second, Marx and Engels's thesis alleges that until the revolution comes, the family will remain as a branch of the state, a keeper of kin and lot, but it will not oversee relations of production, distribution, and power, for that will continue to be based on class. And as the state rises in sync with capitalism, it assumes more significance in what was once the family domain (e.g., educating the young). This is part of the dominance of the state and its power to control working people in order to protect the interests of the privileged.

Finally, as Marx and Engels saw it, the rise of the state directly affects family relations. In protecting the rights of property and weaponry which are predominately controlled by men, the state systematically supports the exploitation of wives and children. Not only does one class acquire power over another, but one person dominates over the rest of the family. The new family arrangement is what Marx and Engels called *father-right,* and it is associated with "the principle of naked authority" within the family. The relationship between husbands and wives, was, to Marx and Engles, the smallest model in which the well-being and development of one group are attained by the misery and repression of another group.

The Frankfurt School

The Frankfurt School is the name given to the privately funded Institute for Social Research established in Frankfurt, Germany, in 1923. It became famous for such scholars in residence as Theodor Adorno, Walter Benjamin, Erich Fromm, Max Horkheimer, Otto Kirchheimer, Leo Lowenthal, Herbert Marcuse, Franz Neumann, and Friedrich Pollock. The whole spectrum of these intellectuals' ideas represents the major development of a version of Marxian theory centering on domination, what has been introduced as critical theory (Agger 1979; Arato & Gebhardt 1987). Initially, the Frankfurt thinkers sought to explain why the proletariat in Western Europe had not united and become revolutionary. The efforts of Frankfurt School members culminated in a theory of domination that included an explanation of how ideological, cultural, and psychological factors penetrate to the core of human personality, averting consciousness away from one's own alienation and ideas about emancipation. One theoretical question of importance was this: What is the link between the social structure and the human psyche (Agger 1979; Arato & Gebhardt 1987; Osmond 1987)? The theoretical creation joined Marxism and Freudian psychoanalysis: from Marxism, an analysis of social structures and their historical conditions; from Freudian theory, the concepts and theorems pertinent to explaining the sociopsychological development of the individual (Held 1980). The combination proved fruitful in establishing the relation between the individual and society.

Interest in Freudian theory among the Frankfurt theorists bears on Frued's insights into repression; as defined by Freud, repression means "the process by which a mental act capable of becoming conscious . . . is made unconscious and forced back into the unconscious system" (1965,351). In brief, Freud unearthed the content of the unconscious, a composite of the interplay between instinctual, biological drives and repressive elements. Freud theorized that every human being is born with animalistic, survivalistic drives, especially for sex and aggression, and unless these drives are rechanneled or curtailed, social order is impossible. Interestingly, Freud (1965) found that individuals with obsessions about hard work or religious dogma, for example, tended to be highly repressed, a fact that led him to suggest that the social is founded on repression.

As Freud saw it, every society must develop within each of its members a conscience that will redirect the inborn drives to more socially acceptable forms; in Freud's words:

> Civilization has been built up, under the pressure of the struggle for existence, by sacrifices in gratification of the primitive impulses, and that it is to a great extent for ever being re-created, as each individual, successively joining the community, repeats the sacrifice of his instinctive pleasures for the common good. (1965,27)

Pleasure is the principle behind the inborn drives, according to Freud. Reaching the adult stage requires passing through developmental stages during early childhood, the stages named in terms of their source of pleasure: oral, anal, genital, and phallic. At any one of these stages, a child might be overcome by trauma and unconsciously repress the experience, a circumstance resulting in the individual having personality disorders later on in life. Thus, the short of Freud's theory is that every member of society is subjected via the family to a process of repression and sublimation that conditions the individual to what is socially acceptable, heightening the "reality principle" so vital to the order of society (Agger 1979, 237–43).

Adorno was an ardent supporter of the Marxist/Freudian synthesis. According to Held (1980), Adorno, as early as 1955, proclaimed that the sociological and the psychological are each unique yet interdependent and, for this reason, a complete analysis of the individual would necessitate an inclusion of the two. The changing relationship of the individual to society, in Adorno's judgment, works like this: "Every society reaches into the individual, but within the individual, it is translated into a language quite distinct from that of everyday life—'the language of the unconscious'" (Held 1980,110). The relationship between the sociological and the psychological is fluid, though the boundary between the two spheres is separate.

One domain that proved to add insight into the relation between the sociological and the psychological was the family. Frankfurt theorists applied their theoretical ideas to the family in an effort to unveil the element of domination in the family. In this section, the theorists to be discussed are the ones whose work is more oriented to showing how the character of the family and its individual members are conditioned by the social organization in which they are rooted; the theorists are Fromm, Reich, Horkheimer and Marcuse.

Erich Fromm had an insight into the relationship between the social structure and the human psyche that was important to the field of social psychology:

> The role of primary formative factors goes to the economic conditions. The family is the essential medium through which the economic situation exerts its formative influence on the individual's psyche. The task of social psychology is to explain the shared, socially relevant, psychic attitudes and ideologies—and their unconscious roots in particular—in terms of the influence of economic conditions on libido strivings. (1932,486)

In "The Method and Function of an Analytic Social Psychology," Fromm (1932) regarded instinctual drives as a biological given subject to modification via the family which he saw as a product of a specific socioeconomic situation; the rundown being, the child, is conditioned by the family, which is conditioned by its class background which is a condition of the social structure. The gist of all this is that social-psychological phenomena are "processes involving the active and passive adaptation of the instinctual apparatus to the socioeconomic situation" (Fromm 1932,486). Adaptation, as understood by Fromm, is simply human instinct adapting to a social reality that is humanly constructed, meaning it is not natural.

With his position on the phenomena of social psychology set forth, Fromm castigated the majority of psychoanalytic works of his time for failing to locate the family within a specific structure. Psychoanalysts had generalized about all families from the families they studied, which were largely from the bourgeois class; and they had taken at face value the structure of bourgeois society, including its patriarchal family. Presenting the social structure in generic terms was made possible, Fromm reasoned, because the investigators were straight-out unaware of their bourgeois bias: "They had turned bourgeois, capitalist society into an absolute; and they more or less consciously believed that it was the 'normal' society, that its conditions and psychic factors were typical for 'society' in general" (1932,484).

Fromm surmised that instinctual drives, conditioned by class, are altered in such a way as to affect the social process, that is instinctual drives are modified by the social process, and vice versa. The interplay between instinctual drives and the social process accounts for ideology in that it explains how the material base is reflected in the human mind—the human psyche is part of the substructure of society. Fromm concluded that "psychoanalysis within historical materialism will provide a refinement of method, a broader knowledge of the forces at work in the social process, and greater certainty in understanding the course of history and in predicting future historical events" (1932,492).

Although Wilhelm Reich was not one of the members of the Frankfurt School, he was one contemporary whose ideas greatly influenced them, especially Horkheimer and Marcuse. As Held (1980, 110–11) points out, the institute's scholars praised Reich for not reducing Marxism to Freudian psychoanalysis, something he accomplished by approaching the social and the instinctual as related yet separate spheres; the approach was adopted by the critical theorists. Reich's attention to the connection between the authoritarian family repression (in this case, sexual inhibitions) and to the larger society was of special interest to the residents at Frankfurt.

In two of his early works, *Character Analysis* (1949) and *The Mass Psychology of Fascism* (1933), Reich gives an explanation of how society shapes the character structure of the individual. The explanation involves exploring the way human instincts are shaped and repressed. His thesis is short and simple: "Every social order creates those character forms which it needs for its preservation" (1980,116). Reich regarded capitalist society, in its patriarchal form, as an authoritarian society and, as such, one in need of individuals who are fearful of and obedient to authority.

The way "acquiescent subjects" are produced begins early in the family when the child is punished for expressing sexual impulses. As Reich explains, "the moral inhibition of the child's natural sexuality, the last stage of which is the severe impairment of the child's genital sexuality, makes the child afraid, shy, fearful of authority, obedient, 'good,' and 'docile' in the authoritarian sense of the words" (1933,30). Crippled is the child's ego and rebellious forces. The fear continues throughout the individual's life, repressing indefinitely "vital life-impulses," thereby causing rigid and reactionary thinking. In short, the child is forced to adapt to authoritarian structure, first in the family, then in the larger society. Reich's way of looking at this is that "the family is the authoritarian state in miniature, to which the child must learn to adapt himself as a preparation for the general social adjustment required of him later" (1933,30). Thus, to Reich, adaptation represents forced conformity.

It was Reich's optimistic belief that in a noncapitalist, nonpatriarchal society, "ascetic sexual ideology" could prevail, making possible many kinds of honest and cooperative human relations. But until there is a change in the existing social order, there will be the same basic process of sexual negation, the same ideology "anchored" in the character structure of the individual, the same authoritarian patriarchy ensuring an authoritarian state and people will continue to oppress and be oppressed. To Horkheimer, Reich's insights were inspiring but in need of further refinement; hence

Horkheimer would engage himself in developing an explanation of the changing structure of the individual and the family.

Probably the most notable critique of the bourgeois family is that of Max Horkheimer. In an essay on authority and the family appearing in *Critical Theory* (1972), Horkheimer sought to show how the relation of individuals to authority in capitalist society is determined by the specific mode of production, which gives rise to character types corresponding to the work process. Horkheimer maintained that the family has a special place in the relationship of influencing the psychic character of the individual:

> The family, as one of the most important formative agencies, sees to it that the kind of human character emerges which social life requires, and gives this human being in great measure the indispensable adaptability for a specific authority-oriented conduct on which the existence of the bourgeois order largely depends. (1972,98)

One of the goals of the bourgeois family is to internalize within the child "submission to the categorical imperative of duty"; hence, adaptability in Horkheimer's book means submission. The submission is perfected each time the child bows down to the superiority of the father, an act infused with "obedience to God." Associating strength with what is loved, the child learns to reason that submission is a moral act. This "training" prepares the child for the authoritarian conditions of life outside the family. However, as Horkheimer stresses, the child submits to the father not out of respect but because the father is stronger, and this is a new condition brought about by the advancement of capitalism. Whereas the father once guided his children through all facets of their lives and had control over his work and everyday life, today human education is mainly offered outside the home. The father is simply one more cog in the wheel in the work world, a man controlled rather than in control, except at home where he reigns as disciplinarian. The outcome is a master of the house who is not honored as much as he is feared.

The family in the Western world has been in decline, according to Horkheimer, ever since the "the growth of large-scale manufacturing and increasing unemployment." The biggest change has been the replacement of the matriarchal system with patriarchy; this change "introduced mankind to class conflict and to the rupture between public and familial life, while within the family the principle of naked authority came to be applied" (1972: 118). The separation of space and time of the work and family world has reduced the father to money earner, the mother to sexual object and domestic specialist, and their children to possessions, social security, and heirs. In early capitalism, the family was a haven from the dehumanization and authoritarianism of the world. In time, though, the public became more powerful and controlling, the private world more powerless and oppressive. In the work place, there is the paycheck but also the competition and the subordination. At home, there is the solitude of domesticity but also, for wife and children, the station of dependency. Consequently, the decline of the family represents to Horkheimer a decline in family functions and individual autonomy. It also represents the larger social order being reproduced within the family.

Herbert Marcuse also endeavored to link human personality and society through Marxian and Freudian concepts, only his goal was different: to present a theory on how to initiate large-scale social transformation through personal radicalism. His position was that repression is a historical phenomenon, "the effective subjugation of the instincts to repressive controls . . . imposed not by nature but by man" (1955,15).

Marcuse argued that while instinctual constraint was initially in response to scarcity, it has been intensified by the hierarchical distribution of goods and labor and now continues in spite of the fact that scarcity is no longer of issue in technologically advanced societies. Today, human beings are subjected to "surplus repression," or repression beyond that which is required to maintain a social group. Instinctual inhibition and restraint are, as Marcuse would have them, factors of domination that come from outside and from within the individual, that is, in accordance with Freud's "reality principle" plus "surplus repression," or the alienation individuals do to themselves. The necessity for heightened repression in mature capitalist societies is to keep humans in high productive gear so that they are "the subject–object of socially useful labor" and steady consumers.

Consumerism includes both true and false needs: "true" means vital needs (i.e., food, clothing, and shelter); "false" refers to needs superimposed on individuals to make them feel gratified; they are repressive needs inasmuch as their content and function are determined by powers over and beyond the individual. The prevalence of false needs is undeniable in a society where individuals find themselves in their commodities; people have come to find their souls in such things as sports cars, designer labels, and dishwashers instead of experiencing the happiness that comes with the development of personal abilities and talents. In Marcuse's opinion, the distinguishing feature of advanced industrial society

> is its effective suffocation of those needs which demand liberation"; what we have instead is "the need for stupefying work where it is no longer a real necessity; the need for modes of relaxation which soothe and prolong this stupefication; the need for maintaining such deceptive liberties as free   competition at administered prices, a free press which censors itself, free choice between brands and gadgets. (1964,7)

The short of it is that human beings believe they are free when in fact they are exploited.

Monopoly capitalism demands adaptation. It needs people who lack zesty character and a zeal for fundamental change, the "one-dimensional" types. Subordination to the economy is seeped into the individual's consciousness through first the family and then the media. Marcuse wrote that "the primal father, as the archetype of domination, initiates the chain reaction of enslavement, rebellion, and reinforced domination which marks the history of civilization" (1955,15). Although Marcuse sees society as still being held together by the libidinal relationship, he also contested that the prevailing forms of social control are technological:

> The means of mass transportation and communication, the   commodities of lodging, food, and clothing, the irresistible output of the entertainment and information industry carry with them prescribed attitudes and habits, certain intellectual and emotional reactions which

bind the consumers more or less   pleasantly to the producers and, through the latter, to the whole. (1964,12)

Technology thus institutes effective forms of social control. Technology is a dominating force behind mass oppression, though it has the potential to improve the human condition qualitatively. Marcuse complained of how, at a time when there is the know-how and materials to free people from want and daily toil, this potential is not realized because of the interests of society's dominant class. And not only are the society's own citizens exploited but so too are human beings abroad, who must suffer deprivation in order that the dominant society may produce and consume an "abundance of wares"; to this, Marcuse shouted "Obscene."

The political force that could change the world and liberate the individual is, assured Marcuse, as basic as a "new sensibility." The sensibility concept stresses how human beings in their everyday lives can cast off the chains of alienation and surplus repression by having new modes of perception and feeling that enhance the aesthetic and the ethical within each person and, ultimately, the world over. Marcuse called for reshaping reason, the way the world is "ordered, experienced, changed." He sought a transformation that "would be nonviolent, nondestructive: oriented on the life-enhancing, sensuous, aesthetic qualities inherent in nature" (1969,67). If Eros (sublimated sexuality) were liberated from surplus repression, then the pleasure principle would be superior to the reality principle, which would create a societal emancipation where work could be creative and relationships nonexploitative.

More Recent Contributors: Poster and Lasch

Mark Poster finds Marcuse and the other Frankfurt theorists lacking a proper conception of the family and, as a consequence, offering a weak link between psychic and social structure. The problem is that the Frankfurt theorists fail to include emotional patterns in their explanations of family structure. In order to correct the flaw, Poster conceptualizes the family as "the place where psychic structure is formed and where experience is characterized in the first instance by emotional patterns" (1978,143).

Poster proposes analyzing the family from these three levels: (1) the psychological level, (2) the family's everyday life and (3) its relation to society. Levels 2 and 3 are supplementary to the first level (1978,143). With the new concept and categories for studying the family, the divergent family structures become more intelligible, that is, it is possible to account for the family's particular psychological patterns, unique experiences, and participation in social institutions.

Under Poster's conceptualization, the family is not primarily an agent of socialization but is, instead, the "social location where psychic structure is most decisively prominent" (1978,143). A study of family structure agreeable to Poster must include Freudian developmental stages (oral, anal, and genital), the pattern of authority and love between adults and children, and identification patterns bonding family members. Poster summarizes his conception of the family as follows: "In summary, the family is here conceptualized as an emotional structure, with relative autonomy, which constitutes hierarchies of age and sex in psychological forms" (1978,155).

In the final chapter of *Critical Theory of the Family* (1978), Poster establishes the family found in today's capitalist society, conventionally called the modern family, as a more recent version of the bourgeois family of mid-nineteenth-century Europe. After examining models of the bourgeois, aristocratic, peasant, and working class families in Europe from the late Middle-Ages to mid-nineteenth century, Poster concludes that the bourgeois family is a "historically distinct phenomenon."

The bourgeois family's notable characteristics include its urban setting, separate spheres between work and home, privatized household, family planning, sexual inhibitions, monogamous marriage, strict sex-role division, rigid child-rearing methods, and emphasis on individualization. The characteristics constitute a "particular emotional pattern which served to promote the interests of the new dominant class and to register in a unique way the conflicts of age and sex" (1978,177). The distinct emotional pattern of the bourgeois family is defined "by authority restricted to parents, deep parental love for children and a tendency to employ threats of the withdrawal of love rather than physical punishment as a sanction," writes Poster (1978,177). The following is a glance at the more prominent characteristics of the bourgeois family.

With the advancement of capitalism, there came to be a separation between work and home, mainly so that men could devote themselves entirely to industry and economy. The separation created a situation in which the public world was regarded as a place of reason and the private a place of emotion, and these distinctions were then projected onto the individual. Men were seen as rational, women as emotional. The bourgeois family world became a world in which outsiders, including authorities, were not free to intervene. Husbands were disciplinarians, providers, and somebodies through their work, women derived their identities and positions in life from their husbands and their major assignment: to raise children.

Bourgeois mothers, expounds Poster, "were not simply to tend to the survival of their children, but to train them for a respectable place in society . . . (and) to create a bond between themselves and the children so deep that the child's inner life could be shaped to moral perfection" (1978,170). Moreover, whatever shortcomings befell her children, the mother was deemed responsible. The formidable assignment in view of Victorian morality and family isolation resulted in the practice of strict child-rearing methods. Mothers gave their full attention to their children's feedings and cleanliness, instilling within the children that what their bodies produced was disgusting and must be controlled and what their bodies could do pleasure-wise via masturbation was horrifying and unacceptable under any circumstance.

The training created ambivalence, love and hate toward one's body and toward one's parents in the drama between desiring bodily pleasure and parental love. Ambivalence deeply internalized within the child attitudes of bourgeois respectability, and for this reason, Poster considered it the emotional core of the bourgeois child. The ambivalence fostered an "autonomous" and disciplined human being, a self-motivated individual prepared for the competition and challenges in a dog-eat-dog world. Autonomy, though, is an illusion. The bourgeois may feel a self-made person, "as the captain of his soul," but in reality, he or she is "the result of complex psycho-social processes" (1978,178).

Poster successfully presents the family as a multilinear, heterogeneous phenomenon. He explains how the family structure includes social and psychological patterns woven from the mass base of society, not modernization. Realized are the many forms family takes under various circumstances. By redefining the family structure away from size toward emotional patterns, Poster is able to elaborate on the unparalleled dynamics of the bourgeois family in the nineteenth century, the predecessor of today's family in the capitalist world.

Like Poster, Christopher Lasch is concerned with the making of the "modern family" in Western Europe and the United States, considering the family's emotional organization along with its size and structure and concluding that domestic life within a bourgeois family system "created psychological conditions favorable to the emergence of a new type of inner-directed, self-reliant personality—the family's deepest contribution to the needs of a market society based on competition, individualism, postponement of gratification, rational foresight, and the accumulation of worldly goods." Where Lasch differs from Poster, and from previous critical theorists, is in his view of the family as a haven under capitalism (1977,4).

The family in the nineteenth century, according to Lasch (1977), was a haven only insofar as the outside world had become more "forbidding." The private domain had not become warmer and cozier but merely an "emotional fortress" forced on individuals by a circumstance that included impoverished work, competitive civil life, and the collapse of communal traditions. And as "the machinery of organized domination" churned onward, it mixed the private with the public, resulting in a domestic poison; hence, the family as a haven was doomed from its onset.

A Paradigm Shift: Feminist Critical Thought

Rejection of the family as a haven under capitalism has also been voiced by feminists such as Nancy Fraser, who writes that families are the "sites of egocentric, strategic and instrumental calculation as well as sites of usually exploitative exchanges of services, labor, cash and sex, not to mention sites, frequently, of coercion and violence" (1987,37). And Jean Bethke Elshtain (1981), while acknowledging that families can be locales of oppression, presses feminists not to forget how under advanced capitalist patriarchy, families are often the one place where the individual can find a semblance of love and security, and moreover express through word

and deed ideas and values that may run counter to those of the state
(e.g., the Mennonite view on war). Such criticism and insights
regarding the family are based on a paradigm that goes beyond the
primacy of orthodox Marxism and Freudianism.

Theoretically progressing from the intellectual tradition of
Marxism and Freudianism, feminist theorists seek a new paradigm
that unites the orthodox and their own ideas about how social reality
is organized via a gender system. The need for the paradigm shift
comes from the inability of Marxist and Freudian theorists to explain
comprehensively the oppression of women universally (Donovan
1986; Tong 1989).

The paradigm shift begins with the work of Marxist feminists,
who agree with their fellow Marxists that capitalism created (1) a
more rigid sexual division of labor, (2) a separation between the
public and the private, and (3) a specialization and hierarchization
of labor, but question the role of domestic labor and women's
placement in the class structure under capitalism.

The issue of domestic labor starts with the limited definition of
production presented in Marxian theory, which trivializes women's
work. From the feminist viewpoint, reproduction is part of production;
accordingly, child-rearing and household activities are historical
aspects of human existence that are located at the center of changes
in the economy (Nicholson 1987). Given the feminists' expanded
version of production, Margaret Benston (1969) claims women
constitute a class of people relegated to the production of simple use-
values within the home and family. Marxist feminists Mariarosa
Dalla Costa and Selma James (1972) argue that under capitalism,
women's work is production in the sense that it creates "surplus
value" and thus should be paid work. Combined, the work of Marxist
feminists redefines notions of productive labor and class as they
relate to the situation of women under capitalism; however, as
socialist feminists charge, Marxist feminists fail to explain the
exploitation of women in precapitalist and postcapitalist societies
(Donovan 1987; Tong 1989).

Socialist feminist agree that women outside capitalism have not
lived free of dominance; patriarchy (i.e., a male-dominated society
where women as women are exploited by men as men) existed long
before capitalism and now exists in Third World countries and
socialist societies, as well as in advanced capitalist societies (Barrett

1980; Jaggar 1983). The mode of women's oppression in pre-and postcapitalist societies is patriarchy, and in capitalist societies it is both capital and patriarchy.

Although class and gender are separate categories, they need not be placed in a separate-sphere feminist model, urges Iris Young, a socialist feminist. Young's defense of a unified-systems theory rests on her idea that the shape of patriarchy is formed by the existing economic system. Under capitalism, patriarchy is manifested in, for example, women's experiences with sexual harassment on the job, low wages in the paid work place, and not being compensated for domestic work.

Thus a material base for patriarchy in a capitalist society has been established by socialist feminists. The general consensus is that while capitalism did not create patriarchy, it enabled it to flourish as a result of the separation of men into the highly valued public realm and women into the trivialized private realm, thereby separating the sphere of social production from the home (Barrett 1980). Under this arrangement, all men in a capitalist society benefit from a sexist ideology that glorifies the traits to which they are socialized, such as competitiveness, rationality, and authority, and are needed for survival in a public world where exchange is the name of the game, while belittling female characteristics, such as nurturance and emotionality and the whole sphere of the private, use-value realm; this stereotypical sexual behavior created via ideological socializtion is, according to Heidi Hartmann (1981), functional to the capitalist system. Given that most of the socialization of children occurs in the home and is done by women, some feminists including Heidi Hartmann and Nancy Chodorow have turned their attention to the process of ideological socialization (Donovan 1987). Chodorow in particular has made a major contribution to our understanding of the process through an integration of Freudian theory with Marxism, thus furthering the earlier work of the Frankfurt School.

Unlike her theoretical predecessors in psychoanalysis, Chodorow (1978) argues that gender differences in a capitalist society are rooted in the psychodynamics of early childhood; the psychic reproduction process, mainly monitored by mothers as a consequence of women being consigned to the private realm, includes shaping, differentially, the personalities of males and females for the con- tinuance of capitalist patriarchy. The developmental process involves mothers identifying more with their daughters than their sons and thus not rejecting their daughters but rejecting their sons at the end of the preoedipal phase. Boys, who are forced to redefine themselves from their mothers in the absence of their idealized fathers, eventually identify themselves in contradistinction to their mothers and all that is feminine. Daughters, in contrast, remain relatively enmeshed with their mothers. As a result, sons develop a sharper sense of distinctiveness or ego boundaries than the daughters, who develop of sense of self that is connected rather than separate to the world. The emotional organization of the sons is thus compatible with capitalist values, whereas the daughters' emotional makeup is best suited for social needs. The process ultimately results in a world in which disjuncture between the sexes prevails. It is a process in which women inadvertently perpetuate their own oppression.

It is Chodorow's belief that primary parenting shared between men and women would result in androgynous emotional organizations. In this event, men would no longer acquire the character traits functional for the capitalist work structure and, presumably, capitalism would wither away. The individual radicalism echoes from Marcuse's lyrics, only Chodorow was not thinking in praxis-terms (Donovan 1986).

Support of Chodorow's ideas about the differential development between the sexes is found in Carol Gilligan's *In a Different Voice* (1982). In the book, Gilligan shares her discovery of how theories of moral development have been constructed by males from data derived almost exclusively from studies of males, and thus the developmental norm has been based on male behavior at the exclusion of women which is why Gilligan initially had difficulty interpreting women's development. Gilligan found that the cornerstone of male development is differentiation, whereas women's begins in relatedness, a reality emerging from early parent/child relations as described by Chodorow. One reflection of the differential discovered by Gilligan is how women and men think differently about morality: When women think about morality, it is in the context of human connectedness, of overlapping relationships and responsibilities. For men, morality is thought of in terms of rights, privileges, conventions, and so on of a hierarchical ordering. Understanding the differential is, according to Gilligan, an important step toward better relations between the sexes and between family members.

For feminists, the focus of their theory is more on sexuality than material conditions with regard to ideological construction (Donovan 1986). And, of course, this is one way in which the feminists differ from the other critical theorists. Yet, like the Frankfurt School theorist Marcuse, feminists believe consciousness raising is a form of revolutionary praxis; this position has been labeled anarchist by Donovan (1986). For example, Carol Ehrlich (1981,114) embraces the anarchist position, which involves people learning "the habits of freedom and equality by attempting to practice them in the present .... The primary means of doing this is through building alternative forms of organization alonside the institutions of the larger society." For Ehrlich and feminists with a social anarchist position, "revolution is a process, not a point in time."

Other feminists with a social anarachist bent have urged, too, that feminists develop the following legitimate forms of praxis: developing alternative arrangements, restructuring work away from alienated labor, and building alternative institutions which includes changing personal relationship (Donovan 1986). An applied version of the praxis is what Nancy Hartsock (1983) calls the feminist standpoint. In Hartsock's (1983,246) words, the feminist standpoint is a perspective and practice derived from women's "experience of continuity and relation with others, with the natural world, of mind with body" as opposed to the "abstract masculinity" to which men are socialized in the capitalist world of commodity exchange. The point is that in order to pull away from oppression, both the institutions of society and the mind of the individual must change (Jaggar 1983).

The critical thought that has arisen from Marx to feminists is in response to the emergence of an authoritarian order in which domination is maintained through controlling consciousness by reproducing at the deepest level of the individual, the values and behavior that serve to maintain capitalist patriarchy. Concern with the sociological and the psychological as two interrelated parts of the relation between the individual and society has shown its strength in demystifying notions about the "naturalness" of the social order. The individual's sense of autonomy and individualiza-tion, for example, have been traced to dimensions of repression within the immediate context of the family, revealing how the individual is coerced into conformity.   And the family, with its hierarchical and authoritarian structure, has been shown to be the site where gender relations are initially structured in addition to being a miniature model of the domination in the larger social order. Critical thinkers have revealed the antagonistic character of social relations in order to identify that which needs to be abolished, an intellectual foundation derived from Marx, Lukacs, and Gramsci. The alternative theorists are not neutral but are driven by the desire to destroy domination, to create a society that can sustain human happiness and dignity for all its members. In a free society, human senses and action would be open to the workings of social relations, and science would have a different presumption, one that starts with the totality of nature. Adaptation would take on the meaning of society, adjusting its materials and myriad resources to meet the needs of the individual so that each person's potential would be fully developed. As Marcuse dreamed, moral and aesthetic needs would become fundamental needs and there would be a "drive toward new relationships between the sexes, between the generations, between men and women and nature" (1969,17); and as many feminists have envisioned, the family in a free society would take on new forms liberated from gender-oppressive features (Tong 1989).

While works by critical thinkers have been helpful in illuminating the dynamics of the emotional structure in the child/parent relationship, little has been said in the critical literature about the emotional structure of the intergenerational relationship once the child has become an adult. I propose an evaluation of the adult child/parent relationship that accounts for the psychological pattern of the family under the current social organization of American society. A focus on the qualitative aspects of the older familial relationship should be fruitful for accomplishing this proposal.

Chapter	2	DIMINISHING AMBIVALENCE

The present-day intergenerational relationship is far from perfect, but equally, it is ages away from disintegration. Contradictions abound within the intergenerational relationship: Baby boomers are disengaged yet bonded, distant yet beside, dishonest yet bona fide, for example, in their relations with their parents. What underscores the special character of the relationship of adult children under advanced capitalist patriarchy is the ambivalence experienced by the offspring long after childhood; adult children are torn between pulls of parental love and personal desires. And in a general structure where love is confused with authority and protection with control, the ambivalence is augmented all the more.

The position of mainstream social gerontology, as addressed earlier in this work, is that adult children should adapt to "modern American life" in order to create a near-perfect intergenerational relationship. As the findings of the study at hand show, this position, established on ideological premises and supported by demographic data, is ill-conceived and thus is an inappropriate response to the problem. Inasmuch as the position might seem reasonable, it is necessary to note that it is laden with ideological overtures and steeped in insensitivities toward the real nature of the intergenerational relationship. If adult children were simply to adapt, they would be conforming to an authoritarian and unjust system that provokes, not soothes, social tensions and individual hardships.

Certainly, what would come to pass would not be closer and more caring intergenerational relationships. More likely, filial adaptation would breed ambivalence to boot, for it would intensify and not diminish the prevailing pulls on the adult children. Why? Because filial adaptation in its complete definition circumscribes adult children to a sexist ideology that tears away the socially defined "masculine" elements in the females and the "feminine" elements in the males. It also serves an economic ideology that cradles opposite social demands, one being personal expression and the other being deference to authority figures. The result would be greater intergenerational discord and further oppression and suffering at both individual and societal levels.

Plainly, prescriptions for filial adaptation are callings for adult children to conform to a way of life specific to a capitalist patriarchical society. In the filial adaptation position, "modern life" is a euphemism for a monopoly capitalism coupled with patriarchy. "Adaptation" promotes conformity and "perfect intergenerational relationships" supports intact hierarchical (including patriarchal), authoritarian relations. This way of life, while beneficial to some, is for the majority alienating and oppressive, suffocating all possibilities for egalitarian relations. Hence filial adaptation is part of the problem behind strained intergenerational relations and therefore is the wrong approach if the genuine goal is progressive relations between the generations.

It is my belief that improvements need to be made in the intergenerational relationship, not because it is a familial relationship, but because it is a human relationship. And this is one major point of contention between myself and mainstream social gerontologists. My concern is with finding ways to improve the human condition, not support the existing social order; the issue to me is how the family arrangement contributes to human suffering as opposed to how it is intricately tied to today's social stability. As far as the adult child/parent relationship goes, my interest lies in instituting a nonauthoritarian relationship. Reforming the intergenerational relationship requires changing the social demands on the individual (not the other way around). In this sense, my approach is radical.

Looking at the familial relationship as a human relationship is significant with regard to a changed, freer society in that it allows for more realistic expectations with respect to the intergenerational relationship. Even under the best of circumstances, the adult child/ parent relationship would not be a perfect relationship; it is a human relationship subject to human imperfections. But the intergenerational relationship could be improved from what it is today, and that is what concerns us here.

By listening to the spoken words of the baby boomers, instead of relying exclusively on demographics and surveys, in trying to piece together the emotional structure of the present-day family, I have come to understand better the social demands obstructing nonauthoritarian, nonhierarchical relations between adult children and their parents in the United States. I am convinced that the problem is a public rather than a private one.

I am also convinced that Marcuse and Chodorow are right in their suggestions that a radical transformation of the individual can initiate a radical change in the larger social order and that social anarchist feminists are right in their notion of social revolution, that is, it is a process, not a point in time. My conviction on radical change lies in my understanding of the intergenerational relationship. Let me explain.

The social demands on the individual in the United States revolve around the needs of a patriarchical, capitalistic system. The demands are extensive, but basically boil down to the need for (1) women to be socially charged and prepared to comfort the emotional world of domesticity, and (2) men to be self-charged and prepared to confront the competitive world of capitalism. Both women and men are socialized to participate heartily in consumerism, to accept hierarchical structures as natural situations, and to acquiesce to authority, which for women also means acquiescing to men. Concisely, the need is for individualization. And, as explained earlier, the individual is introduced to the social demands at home.

With the help of Freud and Poster, we know that individualization is a product of the bourgeois family structure and, thanks to feminists, we know it is also a product that under partriarchy is packaged differently for women and men. The ability for individuals to act on their own individualization is learned through ambivalence. Children, especially daughters, are taught by their parents, most often by their mothers, that what their bodies produce is disgusting and needs to be controlled and that their bodily sensations should not be manually produced. They are also taught that their bodies should not be heard. The sound of urination, defecation, passing gas, belching, and all other natural bodily sounds are deemed despicable and offensive to others. Humanness must not be heard. Children learn that they must choose between their bodily gratifications and parental affection which deeply instills within the children the need for mastering and silencing their bodies which, when internalized in the unconsciousness, fosters appropriate social attitudes of respectability, thereby generating the needed autonomy and acquiescence so vital for the continuation of advanced capitalism. And for daughters, the lesson is magnified, thereby helping to sustain patriarchy.

Continued throughout the children's lives, well into their adulthood, are the parental lessons on respectability by sex, though geared toward other personal dimensions of the children, such as hair length, style of clothing, career choice, selection of spouse, child-rearing, and location of residence. Each lesson reinforces the ambivalence, thereby sustaining the individualization. The dynamics of power and domination are continually reinforced as parents attempt to control their children's respectability as well as the terms of the intergenerational relationship (e.g., defining to the children what topics are open for discussion). Yet what is also propagated by the reinforcement is strain in the intergenerational relationship. What would make for better relations between the generations would be the abandonment of such social demands. The formula for nonauthoritarian, nonhierarchical relations between adult children and their parents is elementary: Abolish domination from the family structure. In that domination is something we exercise on ourselves by participating as autonomous beings in an oppressive system, the formula is feasible, but in that the mass base of exploitation is rooted in the ideology of gender division coupled with the larger social relations under advanced patriarchal capitalism, it is problematic. In other words, we can change our immediate environment but without transcending content; that is, changing the larger oppressive structure, liberation will not go beyond successful adaptation to the existing establishment. A reminder that personal struggles are also political ones.

Intertwined are the personal and the political, and herein lies the key to both individual and social emancipation As Marcuse lectured, the emancipation of human consciousness is the basis for radical transformation of reality: "Without it, all emancipation of the senses, all radical activism, remains blind, self-defeating" (1969,132). Recall, too, that consciousness raising as a form of revolutionary praxis is the dominant assumption in contemporary feminist theory (Donovan 1986). Given that the liberation of the personal and the political have in common the emancipation of human consciousness, the requisite to change human consciousness seems paramount. And what better place to free human consciousness than at the location where it is most directly and profoundly experienced, namely, in the home.

If improved relations between the generations is truly desired, then the effort must be to dismantle authoritarian, hierarchical relations inside the home with the intent of doing the same outside. In short, the demand is to construct a better social totality via consciousness building, developing a way of thinking about new possibilities for the human condition that are nonoppressive, thereby transforming more than merely modifying the structure. The goal requires, in the words of Marcuse, "a total reconstruction of the technical and natural environment" (1969,30), and in the words of Hartsock, "creating a situation in which thinking and doing, planning and routine work, are parts of the work each of us does; it requires creating a work situation in which we can both develop ourselves and transform the external world" (1981,118). Expectedly, the liberating alternative would result in a different way of life, with different sex relations, different work relations, different forms of economic distribution, different goals and values, different notions about morality, and, of issue here, different familial relations.

Converting to new relations in the home begins with an awareness of the damage caused by authoritarian, hierarchical relations and then a deliberate effort to avoid the interactions and attitudes that feed into the oppressive structure. In the pages to come, I illuminate how the present social organization of American society damages the adult child/parent relationship.

Improvements in the intergenerational relationship demand abolition of the authoritarian, hierarchical structure. Realistically, though, parents of today's adult children probably will not be receptive to efforts to transform the structure of the present-day, older family. Baby boomers, who sang songs about revolution and satisfaction during their teen years and later engaged themselves in breaking traditions, are more likely candidates for implementing real change between themselves and their children if, of course, they have a longing for more harmonious intergenerational relations.

Out of my interviews came clues to ways of transcending authoritarian, hierarchical relations between children and their parents; basically, these narrow down to "support" for and an "attitude of equality" between family members. The excerpts to follow merely represent cases in which the baby boomers reported why they felt close to their parents and/or what they considered to be the more favorable aspects of their immediate intergenerational relationships. Although the baby boomers were merely describing that which pleased them about their parents, revealed is how ambivalence in the adult child can be diminished somewhat when the parents are willing openly to support their child and regard their child as an individual. For example, Hannah said that she and her parents preserve a more open relationship with one another because her parents have always been supportive of her and her siblings:

> They [her parents] are supportive of all of us [siblings]. In that supportiveness, that makes me more open or more willing to be open . . . so there is an intuitive understanding. It's not always verbally communicated.

Hannah finished the interview by telling me how it is that she and her parents are able to maintain a friendship:

> One of the reasons my parents and I have always been able to maintain a friendship as well as they're still my parents . . . and I still respect them and such . . . is their ability to see a child as they are, who they are and let go and let the child move into the world.

Similarly, Leanne, a thirty-five year old bank employee who lives with her parents in a northeastern city, spoke about respect and friendship in her interview:

> We [she and her parents] have our arguments, but generally we treat each other as equals and as thinking people. Then, we have opinions, and they don't always agree, but we seem to respect each other's ideas . . . . I think we are friends in addition to being parents and child.

Leanne defined her relationship with her parents as close and one in which her parents have always been very supportive of her: "I have always felt that there was a very stable, caring—I think religion enters into that—knowing that you have tremendous support at home." Plus, Leanne felt that she and her parents share similar feelings about strong family ties and that this, combined with the mutual respect, the support, and the shared religious beliefs, has strengthened the familial bond.

Hannah and Leanne have emphasized the importance of adult children and their parents reacting to each other as equals. When parents refuse to accept their children as they are, to let go of them, or to see them as "thinking people," they are reiterating their dominance (and insecurities) over their children and, unknowingly, reinforcing ambivalence within their offspring. The subtle yet powerful dispatch says, "You, the child, are not my equal. And, if you want my approval, you must comply with my wishes, even if that means going against your inner passions. The choice is yours." In Hannah's and Leanne's cases, their parents have avoided this tactic, and the result has been two adult child/parent relationships characterized by mutual respect and friendship.

Parental support is still forthcoming for Shira, a graduate student in fine arts at a college in upstate New York:

> I certainly couldn't go back to graduate school at this point in my life if they [her parents] weren't willing to help me . . . . I would also say because they have been so supportive of me, that that makes me feel close to them. And, of course, they're my parents which is inexplicable.

Again, feeling close is tied to parental support, which signals an appreciation for what the adult child is trying to accomplish with her life—even if that is to become an artist—and a respect for the individual regardless of sex, age, and so forth. In another case, the daughter has chosen to be a minister, and today, the parent continues to give Linda plenty of moral support:

> I've been a minister for the past five and a half years. And, when I first went into it, I had to deal a lot with my own need to be approved of by my father. I probably learned most of my theology from my father, so I was always worried about what he was thinking. But now,

> I've seen enough support from him and felt confident
> enough in myself, that even if I don't agree with him, I
> don't care [says this with a laugh].

Linda has brought out an important point that is about the difference
between parents teaching their children and dictating to them, the
former being a nonauthoritarian approach, the latter authoritarian.
Although Linda learned much of her theology from her father, she
is free in her role as adult daughter to express and exercise her own
beliefs around her father without fear of parental retribution. Ambivalence is eased. The child has learned theology, the parent has
learned to accept his child as an individual, and the result is a close,
relatively egalitarian relationship between child and parent.

Being able to speak one's mind openly, to relate to parents as
friends, was also mentioned by Mark, a high school teacher who
grew up in Seattle, Washington:

> How a parent/son relationship can blossom into a
> friendship, as peers, is what has happened over the years
> . . . . You never quite escape the fact that they're your
> parents, but it's nice to be able to relate to them as
> friends, as adults . . . . I think in terms of letting go,
> they've been real good about supporting us.

And when I asked Mark if he had any ill feelings toward his
parents, this is what he said:

> No. There are some things as an adult you can look back
> and look at your parents as adults, as peers, there are a
> couple of things, but I've always been able to talk to
> them about problems . . . If I thought my mom was
> wrong, I could tell her that . . . [and with his dad]. I have
> been able to raise questions.

Mark's comments underscore how crucial it is for parents to be
supportive of their adult children and to let them speak to them in an
open fashion. Parents can take a nonauthoritarian, nonhierarchical
stance that does not feed into adult child ambivalence. The result can

be, as inferred from Mark's case, friendship between the adult child and the aging parents.

The examples given thus far have mainly focused on support and and respect given by the parents to the baby boomers when the children were adults. A few baby boomers, however, emphasized the presence of parental support and egalitarian ideals in the intergenerational relationship during their childhood years. One baby boomer, Les, had this to say about support and equal treatment in the home:

> My parents would always refer to us as family, and we were very conscious of equal treatment of the children and we all got quite a bit of support for the things that we did, myself included. What they wanted most was that our lives would be easier than theirs and that we did the things that we wanted to do.

Caring most about the well-being of the children was also important to Rex's parents. Rex is now an art professor living in upstate New York, but he grew up in St. Paul, Minnesota, the son of a woman who worked as a housewife and a man who was a liquor salesman. In Rex's words, his parents were "really cool" because "they would be real supportive, but they didn't have any idea for a goal for me, which was great!" Furthermore, his parents were more concerned about him and less concerned about keeping up with the Joneses, Rex's closing comment:

> They were really nice people . . . I think I probably had a great childhood . . . . I'd always do terribly in school . . . there was never any instance when my parents told me that wasn't good enough . . . which is really cool . . . . so they were more concerned about me and less concerned about [others] . . . in other words, they wanted their kids to do good but they didn't think, "Well, we should do this and this and this because all of our friends are having kids who are doing this, and this and that.

Parents gave their support in a variety of ways. One was to attend the athletic events of their children and then not criticize them if they lost; this is the background of John, a carpenter at a college in the northeast who has two brothers:

> They supported anything we ever did. We weren't spoiled. But, they backed us up at whatever we did, they really did . . . . They went to all our matches, all our meets, all our games, but they never . . . said a word, whether how good you did. Well, if you did good they said something, but if you did bad they said, "Oh you guys had a bad game." They never tried to tell us what to do.

Today, John's mother is dead, but his father is living. Their relationship seems close. John enjoys visiting with his father: "It's just fun to go down and just talk and lean on him . . . it's a relief."

Finally, a baby boomer by the name of Ed works in the machine shop at a small, private college in New York. He said he felt very close to his parents, especially his dad, and always found it easy to get their approval:

> I think that deep down I wanted their approval, but they gave it so easy that . . . you didn't have to work for their approval . . . even like with school work where they wanted us to do the best, as long as they thought we were trying, they didn't get on our case . . . . I think they did a very good job [of child rearing] . . . . I find it very hard to be as good as they were.

And Ed's last words in the interview:

> They both believed in hard work and doing their share, which I do . . . and being proud of what you do as far as work goes . . . . I'm trying to impress on my kids that there's nothing wrong with helping your neighbor and not charging them ten bucks.

Ed's parents taught him to try to do his best, to be proud of himself, and to care about other people in the world, lessons that his parents gave to him as guides for a strong self-esteem and sense of community. These lessons resulted in one more thing: a close intergenerational relationship.

The parents of Rex, John, and Ed spent less time comparing their children's placement to other children's and more attention to recognizing the individual efforts and interests of their children, a fact that helped relieve some ambivalence of the baby boomers early on in the intergenerational relationship and ended in good familial feelings. Still, the proposition remains that the intergenerational relationship could be much better if only the authoritarian and hierarchical aspects of it were eliminated to a much greater degree than in the cases mentioned thus far.

While the above interviews have given us some insights into the importance of parental support and egalitarian attitudes, they have not shown exactly how the present-day family can transcend authoritarian relations, mainly because the examples presented are of families where socialization has been, in the main, under a patriarchal, capitalist society. If we wish for greater improvements in our families and our larger social structure, then we must consciously set as our goal the demise of oppressive relations. The means to achieve our goal, as elucidated by critical thinkers and dealt with in this book, involves a major restructuring of the socialization of our children and the organization of our societal institutions.

Left to explain is the strain in the adult child/parent relationship. I call attention to the larger social forces influencing the adult child/ parent relationship in the United States. My analysis is aimed at answering the following questions: What are the sources of the strain in the intergenerational relationship? Are the sources of the strain related to the character of the work process under advanced capitalist patriarchy? Are they rooted in the emotional structure of the family? Answering these questions requires accounting for both the sociological and psychological aspects of the family; in short, it requires a critical theory perspective.

The task at hand is a qualitative examination of the intergenerational relationship with the issue being the relation between the family and the larger social order. My analysis explores the emotional structure of the older family and how it is intertwined with structures outside the home. It builds upon the model of the family structure presented by feminists, Poster, and earlier critical theorists. Accordingly, I believe that the family in the United States tends to follow the basic structural features and emotional patterns of the "bourgeois" family, a product of capitalist patriarchy. Consequently, I underscore the oppressive arrangement in the family and other human relations in American society, particularly those surrounding authority and sexual differentials.

Responses surrounding the strain in the intergenerational relationship are divided into five categories derived from open-ended questions presented to the baby boomers. The categories are (1) communication, (2) acceptance, (3) parental control, (4) traditional family dynamics, and (5) forgiveness. Each is examined by chapter, beginning with Chapter 3 and the category of communication.

Chapter	**3**	THE COMMUNICATION PROBLEM

Much of the strain in the adult child/parent relationship can be traced to a lack of communication between the generations. The communication problem is one that originates during the younger family stage and continues into the children's adult years. It consists of parents keeping information from their children, being unable or uncomfortable about discussing personal matters with their children, and not allowing their children to question or express opinions different from their own. It also consists of adult children not confiding in their parents, not expressing to their parents their inner thoughts and feelings, not telling their parents about many aspects of their lives—keeping communication at such a superficial level that their parents do not know them as individuals.

"It's none of your business!"

The baby boomers learned very early on that matters of the "parent world" were matters that their parents would not explain to them, for they were things the children should not know. A clear distinction was made between the "parent world" and the "children world," and the goings on in the "parent world" were for the most part none of the children's business (whereas what went on in the "children world" was their parents' business). It was not uncommon for baby boomers to be left in the dark about human sexuality, family finances, their parents' feelings, or their parents' marital problems.

The fact that parents were exclusive keepers of knowledge placed the young baby boomers at a disadvantaged position in the home. Without ample knowledge, the youngsters could not make sound decisions for themselves or make sense of the world around them. It made them dependent on their parents. Jill, a daughter of divorced parents who spent most of her childhood years in the

Southwest and now lives in Oregon and is twice divorced and raising three kids of her own, had what she believed to be a nervous breakdown at the time she was eight years old, because her parents refused to explain to her (and her siblings) the reason(s) for their divorce and its extenuating consequences:

> I was always quite upset with the way my parents handled their divorce with us children. Everything was kept hush, hush. Nothing was explained. It was just understood that we weren't supposed to understand, we would at a later time. And, we were shuffled back and forth between homes, in and out of courts, and I even lived with my grandparents for three years of my life . . . During the time spent with my grandmother, I actually believe I had a nervous breakdown when I was eight years old.

Jill would later say, in response to having ill feelings toward her parents, that while she loves her parents deeply, yes, she has some ill feelings toward them, in part because of the way they handled their divorce, in part because of the time her mother was totally unfair, in part because of her father's irresponsibility toward the children after he left the home, and to a great extent because of the inability of her parents to appreciate her need for better understanding between the family members, especially between herself and her mother. As Jill pleads:

> She [Jill's mother] never could understand why it was important that I be understood. That I felt is was important to understand her just to maintain my own sanity. And I love her, I love her deeply and I love my father, too. And I always will.

Jill's childhood situation stems from the hierarchical structure in the present-day family, which is mirrowed in the larger social structure. Both in and out of the family, knowledge is power: Who has the knowledge has the power to determine the destiny of oneself and of others; knowledge is well guarded by the powerful in our society (Collins 1975).

Within the present-day family, parents have the knowledge and thus the power. Controlling information in the home is a way of reinforcing parental authority, even if it means causing childhood distress. This pattern of controlling information is paralleled in the workplace and other structures outside the home where individuals are confronted with conditions that have been determined by people higher up, who have the necessary information to make "important decisions."

Both inside and outside the home, those who must oblige to the higher authority are neither invited to participate in the decision-making process nor provided the information that would benefit them in better understanding their current situation. Lack of information places the children and the common people in subordinate positions to persons higher up, which can contribute to their experiencing feelings of insecurity and alienation. It also contributes to misunderstandings and tensions between the family members and between the many groups in society.

While most baby boomers did not reach the point of a "nervous breakdown," many were affected by how little their parents revealed to them about life in general, a fact that to this day causes resentment. One thirty-five-year-old baby boomer who grew up in Cleveland, Ohio, remarked that much of the "ill will" she feels toward her parents today stems from their "closed-mouthed" approach during her formative years, which, as she sees it, resulted in later years in her both doubting her self-worth and being unprepared for adulthood.

In other instances, the secrecy led to conflict between mothers and teenage daughters. Why? Because mothers, left alone much of the time while their husbands were away attending business, were unhappy with their marriages, but instead of saying so, took out their unhappiness on their daughters. Karen, a potter who is the wife of a schoolteacher and the daughter of a homemaker and an executive of a major corporation living in New England, explained:

> I just had a real hard time with my mother . . . We had
> a rough time when I was in high school. She was having
> a hard time. My dad traveled a lot, so there was all this
> stuff she was going through...so I got a lot of that
> sadness . . . . She [mother] was depressed and having a

hard time with Dad. And taking it out on me. And she [mother] talks about it now.

The ill feelings Karen felt toward her mother lasted some ten to twelve years into her adulthood and were not addressed until she sought professional counseling as a young adult because of "attacks, anxiety attacks and phobias" she was experiencing after her first boy friend broke up with her. Through counseling, it was discovered that Karen's insecurities stemmed back to the "rough time" she had with her mother during her teen years. Still, in this instance (as in most), there continues to be a lack of open communication betweem the generations, as Karen testifies: "I hold back about things I really want to talk to them [her parents] about, especially [her mother]." For the most part, Karen has worked through her ill feelings and, as she put it: "I don't harbor a lot of resentment, though there was a time when I did." The child/parent relationship has grown stronger since Karen has been away from home, has lived through some experiences at a distance of several states from her parents, and has sought counseling. Now, as an adult, Karen feels close to her parents. The experiences of Karen and others like her have their origin in the separation of work and home, which traditionally has separated the sexes, belittled the feminine and the needs of females, and encouraged a public world based on impersonal exchanges and a private world based on personal exchanges. In an authoritarian, hierarchical structure, openness is problematic. When impersonal exchanges are experienced in the public place, feelings are less damaged than in the home environment where the expectation is that emotions will be expressed and assuaged. But when the family structure is authoritarian and hierarchical, fulfillment of the emotional at home is not forthcoming, as was true with Karen and her mother, an example of the rough reality of parental authority and patriarchy.

The emotional component of the intergenerational relationship was often kept at a distance, which, to this day, invokes a feeling of anger in some adult children. Meredith, a therapy director at a hospital who is the adult child of an executive secretary and an engineer in North Carolina, said, "They [her parents] hardly gave to me emotionally as a child, and I have anger about that." Meredith has chosen not to marry and have children of her own, a decision she feels is partially based on the this missing emotional element from her childhood years. In explaining why she did not feel close to her parents, Meredith said that in her family, "feelings weren't discussed and talked about"; moreover, feelings are still not discussed today though Meredith wishes they were:

> I've tried to open up discussions with my mother, particularly, just because I'm more comfortable with her and pretty much got shot down . . . I was upset about that . . . . I'm working through that in terms of accepting she hasn't changed, that I've been changing and she hasn't changed. I shouldn't have any reason to expect her to change, so I need to be realistic about that. But that's hard because I would like to be able to relate to her in a different way and it is so difficult.

This "It's none of your business" mentality among the baby boomers' parents represents nothing less than the mentality in the larger social order, which defines privilege through authority and inferiority through dependence. In short, manifestation of the mentality is one way parents ensure a position of dominance over their children. Like the powerless outside the home, many baby boomers have found themselves at different points in their lives confronting authority figures (their parents) who control information that is vital to their destiny, self-worth, and understanding of those with whom they closely associate, the stuff of alienation. Given the sanctity of family privacy, the baby boomers were rarely successful in obtaining the desired information from outside sources. While withholding information secures dominance, it also serves to heighten emotional instability and promote low self-esteem among dependents—not to mention social conflict. This state is worsened within the home when all the other traditional, patriarchal mechanisms are in place (e.g., the isolation and loneliness of the mother).

"Cut that out!"

On the reverse side, baby boomers, while children at home, were not encouraged by their parents to express their thoughts and feelings, particularly those that ran contrary to what their parents believed to be right or proper. In most cases, the baby boomers were not free, as children living under their parents' roofs, to speak their minds. If they did, they were subjected to such ridicule from their parents as "Don't talk back to me!" "So you have all the answers?" "Who are you to question what I say?" "Getting a little big for your britches, eh? "Cut that out, I don't want to hear it!" A thirty-six-year-old bank employee who lives with her parents outside Albany, New York, said, "As a child you learn to accept what was told to you or at least not to project your own ideas if you didn't agree with them [your parents]." Being an open child had its price, according to Jill, the baby boomer from Oregon:

> I was quite an open child. I was the kind who always said what was on my mind regardless of the situation. They [her parents] didn't like me because of it. If I thought they were doing wrong, I told them so, and I would often get punished for it, but that didn't deter me from telling them what I thought. If they were doing something to me that I didn't think was right, I usually tried to remove myself from the situation. There were times that I was punished for that as well.

The inability of many of the baby boomers to be frank with their parents at a young age has sometimes carried over into the older relationship, and this is something that pains many of the baby boomers. An elementary school teacher named Ellen, who grew up in the San Francisco Bay area, said that the worst experience she remembers having with her parents was when she decided to be honest with them on a trip home from college by telling them about "sleeping" with her boy friend. In disapproval, Ellen's father demanded that the boy friend leave the house and never come back and then proceeded to call her a "slut" and threaten to discontinue financially supporting her college education. Ever since the incident, Ellen has not disclosed information to her parents about her relationships with men.

Over the past eight years, Ellen has been living with a man (they were married last year), and for the first six years of the relationship, her parents would not acknowledge her companion, even though Ellen wanted to talk about him to her parents. Consequently, there was a big part of who she was and what she was doing that was not discussed with her parents, a loss deeply felt by Ellen:

> I just thought that was pretty hard-headed of them, and I also felt they were were cutting themselves out of my life really because how could I share with them when they would exclude the most important person to me at this time in my life which I've chosen to make my partner. So, those were ill feelings that lasted for a long time, which I haven't forgiven them [her parents].

In spite of the ill feelings, Ellen still feels close to her parents, mainly because of shared activities:

> I care very much about them [her parents] . . . .the reason I think I like my parents and feel close in some way is because we always did a lot of things together as a family . . . And so even though as an adult I've developed values which are not only different but critical of their values, we still like to see each other and do things together and like each other on that level.

The ill feelings experienced by Ellen and other baby boomers are not about broken familial bonds but about the inability to be heard when their subjects do not suit their parents, prominent persons in their lives. To simplify, the ill feelings are about oppression and submission to authority. The content of conversation is dictated by parents from day 1. Children who wish to be interwoven into their parents' lives learn that they must submit to their parents' authority, a reality that forces ambivalence on adult children in that they must select between the powerful forces of parental affection and personal freedoms. This is the consequence of a structure in which children are regarded as subordinate and parents as dominant.

On another level, the baby boomers have purposely limited self-disclosure to their parents because it has enabled them to maintain a semblance of autonomy. For example, a college professor said she had never confided in her mother, because her mother was "not very comfortable with strong senses of emotion in any way." Furthermore, this person did not volunteer information to her father, a

psychiatrist (who was more interested in being involved in her life
and more perceptive than her mother of her "emotional status"), for
it allowed her a small degree of autonomy from him. The autonomy
factor is also the reason Jill keeps phone calls to her mother at a
minimum:

> I call [Mom] I would gather around once every three
> months, not real often, and the reason being is because
> I enjoy being away. She's [her mother] a very dominat-
> ing-type personality. And the more she knows about
> your life, the more she wants to take control of it and tell
> you how to run it. So, it's better just to stay distant.

Restraint typified the atmosphere within the childhood homes of
the baby boomers, and in some cases it has prevailed to this day.
Freedom to express opinions and emotions, the willingness to
engage parents in life's details have been nipped by the power of
parental authority. The "Cut that out" notion echoes the arrangement
in the larger social structures where authority is one-directional,
downward. Just as workers under a capitalist system traditionally
have not been allowed to bring the human element into work
relations or to speak freely about their condition to their superiors for
fear of retribution, baby boomers have faced an environment in
which they were coerced by their parents to refrain from individual
thought and action that undermined the parents' absolute authority.
About the only degree of independence allotted to the employed is
keeping to themselves, not letting higher rank know too much about
them. Like the working people of this country, offspring have found
that they can preserve a small amount of autonomy by holding back
bits of information about themselves from their parents. Parental
authority is protected, and autonomy too, while the closeness
between parents and children is not. The act began years ago; the
affects are lifelong.

"Don't say a word!"

Some incidents are known as "family matters," and these are not to
be discussed in or out of the home. Everyone understands them, no
one talks about them. "Them" being such things as Tommy's drug

problem, the time Suzie was caught by dad having sex on the sofa with her boy friend, the abortion, father's affairs, mother's drinking, a family suicide, and the like. They are incidents that would create a ghastly scene if someone in the family were stupid enough to mention them. By not talking about the "undesirables," the family basically denies their existence. Meredith told me that her father, who suffers from acute depression, had a mental breakdown when she was nineteen years old. This is how she and her family have reacted ever since his problem: "I reacted like the rest of my family did, by denying it, which wasn't very healthy. The family has not talked about his emotional problems at all..." Ellen, the schoolteacher, in describing a scene of some eighteen years ago when her father went into a tizzy after learning she was having sex with her boy friend, said, "That was really awful, and, nobody ever talked about it again, and I rarely mention [the boy friend's] name."

The "Don't say a word!" posture in the home is a copy of the one used outside the home to cover up tensions, abuses, and failures. These children learned at home that certain realities are shocking to people on the outside, a most appropriate lesson for surviving as an adult in a society where what counts is the facade of decency, not decency itself. If it takes denial to keep the organization, be it the family, the Ford Motor Company, or the FBI, appearing "respectable" to outsiders, then fine, all is well.

And everyone knows it is best not to talk about the faults of the establishment, so the internal conflicts, the sexual harassment, the racial discrimination, the abuses of the safety and hazardous regulations, the fraud, the corruption, the mistreatment of minorities and workers, and so on are just not discussed. No one wants to admit that something is wrong with the organization to which they belong. Interactions in the organization stay at a superficial level, for what matters is not the person as a human being but the person as a status. In order to keep peace, many subordinates simply keep their mouths shut, even when they know they are right.

"How's the weather, dear?"

Lack of communication beyond the superficial level is one of the main characteristics of the intergenerational relationship discussed by the baby boomers in this study. The following quote by Meredith summarizes the sentiment shared by many of the participants:

> When I think about the emotional component to our relationship, there's not a lot of intimacy. I'm not comfortable telling either of my parents my feelings or sharing the real deep aspects of my life. The surface things, the superficial things, are fine.

An emptiness exists in the intergenerational relationship. While many adult children and their parents can talk about such things as "We've been having rain for several days now," "How about those Mets?" or "Mrs. Simmons stopped by today," few can engage in substantive conversations about their personal lives. Michael, the son of a homemaker and a retired college professor, felt disheartened that he, a professional with children himself, did not have anything profound to say to his parents while visiting them:

> In a way when I go out on these visits [to his parents] . . .I feel a little guilty that I don't have something memorable, deep, soul exposing or whatever to say to them, but I don't. And, it just may be that there isn't a whole lot to say or maybe that there have been a lot of years of talking at the surface and not explaining a lot of what's going on.

A similar comment about talk with his mother was voiced by Dan, a sign painter who now lives in Portland but who grew up in Yonkers, New York, and is the son of a housewife and a retired postal carrier now living in Florida:

> We, my mom and I, talk, but it's, it's sort of kept on a superficial level. She's concerned about me, of course, and I really love her. But, I don't talk to her a whole lot about my personal life. I confide in her only up to a certain level.

In response to why he answered positively about having ill feelings toward his father, Dan said,

I wish we would have had a much better communication
. . . . I accept my dad which I think is a horrible place to
be because where I accept him . . . I wish we would have
both been more understanding with each other, so that
we had communication that was more beneficial for
both of us.

And another example of the communication problem comes
from the Cathy, an editor and mother of two boys who lives in New
York, who complained about how she and her parents did not know
each other as individuals. The down side to Cathy's not knowing her
parents aside from their parental roles and their not knowing her
inner thoughts and feelings is that Cathy does not feel close to her
parents. Cathy realizes that she cannot change her parents, so she is
doing her best to try to understand them in order to achieve a sense
of intimacy.

The feeling that parents just do not know you as an individual is
fairly common among the baby boomers. Some baby boomers said
that their parents could not, would not, or thought they did but did
not understand them. The communication problem is frustrating for
many baby boomers, who would like their parents to know them
better but know in their hearts that this will never happen because
their parents are not interested in knowing them, other than as "our
children."

Lack of self-disclosure on the part of parents was another
common complaint voiced by the baby boomers. One man, a potter,
married to a physician, who lives in upstate New York and had just
become a father, decided to ask his parents (on their two-week visit
from Oklahoma to see their newborn granddaughter) about their
lives before they were married. Tom, the baby boomer, was merely
trying to get to know his parents as individuals, but his question,
"What did you do before you were married?" was dismissed by this
response from his dad: "Once you're a family man, that's it, that's
all you are." Discussion closed.

Tom, Cathy, and the other mentioned participants felt that their
parents had slammed shut the door to a more intimate intergenerational
relationship. Discussing the personal, expressing emotion, knowing
parents and having parents know them as people rather than as
statuses, these were the desires of these baby boomers that went

unfulfilled. This structure of impersonalization, while a hindrance to close relations between baby boomers and their parents, has prevailed within the home and the outside world, keeping the dominant and the subordinate in their appropriate places. Authority rests on power and part of power is grounded in remoteness: Too much self-expression would undermine the vantage point of the persons higher up, be they parents, bosses, or officials. Remember, knowledge is power.

Self-expression and sharing the personal are keys to intimate relations, yet they were frequently absent from the relationships under study. Many baby boomers and their parents relate to one another according to status: "You're the child, I'm the parent," therefore, "You should behave this way and I should behave that way." The thought that the two are equals, "I'm an individual and so are you" and "How you behave is unique to you and how I behave is unique to me," escaped most of the family members. Thinking narrowed to statuses and appropriate roles, which also governs other social relations, is crucial for upholding an authoritarian, hierarchical structure, not to mention furthering stereotypes in American society. Succinctly, superficial conversation is a means for securing the current social order.

"It's not important, Mom and Dad!"

In order to keep peace with their parents, some baby boomers simply avoid disclosing too much information about themselves. For example, Ellen said in the interview that she does not confide in her parents about her values and politics:

> I do not confide many or most of the details of my life to my parents. I think we have some very different values and they wouldn't understand some of the ways I lead my life. They would certainly disagree with my political issues and points of view that I hold.

Besides withholding the whole picture of their lives from their parents, some baby boomers maintain intergenerational harmony by avoiding discussions they know will upset their parents; this is especially challenging for baby boomers whose parents are very opinionated or very emotional, as a homemaker in Conneticut noted:

He's [her father] very opinionated, very strong ideas
and not very open to any other people's ideas or thoughts.
He's very hot tempered. It's hard to talk to him about
anything without him getting quite upset . . . . My
father's not the kind of person you can discuss things
with. So, I would talk to my mother, but my mother gets
emotional and upset and I almost feel like I don't want
to tell her anything that's going to make her life uncomfortable or upset her.

Baby boomers who live great distances from their parents tend
to be more reluctant than children living near their parents to engage
in intergenerational confrontation. The attitude is,"We don't see or
talk with each each other that often, let's not spoil the visit with an
argument." A forty-year old self-employed woman named Patricia,
who grew up in New York but moved to Oregon after completing
graduate school, described the special effort as "party manners":

Because I've lived such great distance for the past ten
years from my family, and we weren't around each
other a whole lot, the times we talked on the phone there
was less of that [arguing] . . . when you don't talk to
somebody [except] for half an hour on the phone, it's
easy to be on best behavior, party manners.

Patricia went on to explain that she felt she is able to possess
some inner harmony for the basic reason that she lives across the
country from her parents. The bottom line in all these cases is that
the baby boomers feel that familial harmony is more important than
expressing to their parents what they truly think and feel. It is sort of
an honest/dishonest approach that works to keep intergenerational
relations as warm and cozy as possible. The "honest but dishonest
relationship" is about acquiescing to convention. In both the private
and the public realms, individuals are unwilling to challenge authority
for fear of retribution: Children do not wish to be cut out of their
parents' lives, the employed do not wish to lose their jobs, and
citizens do not wish to be ostracized from their country. Instead of
giving honest accounts of their needs and desires, people limit their
presentations to that which authority figures in their lives wish to
hear. They keep to themselves those values and opinions that run

contrary to those who are in power. Deference is shown to authority figures for the sake of sustaining social harmony. In both realms, a semblance of inner harmony is possible by a physical distancing between the underlings and those who seek to control their lives. In the case of adult children, the fear of retribution, the willingness to fluff facts and feelings, and the deliberate distancing in regard to parents are expressions of ambivalence, the pulls between parental love and personal longings. The end result, at home and at large, is that the individuals, willingly or not, are succumbing to subordinate positions via restraint, as well as learning where they fit into society's hierarchical structures.

In short, I believe that relations within the home reflect and reinforce the authoritarian and hierarchical relations within the larger social order. Earlier critical theorists said that the present-day family in capitalist society is the one realm in which emotion is still central to human relations. Later, Lasch would qualify that the home has never been an absolute haven. The last word on the subject has been presented by critical feminists, who have said that present-day families are locations of oppression. I think, much like Elshtain, there is truth in what all the critical theorists have said. As patriarchal capitalism has advanced, the emotional component in the family has weakened and familial relations have become more exploitative. While family relations resemble the larger oppressive relations under monopoly capitalism, they are still among the rare sites where warmth and emotion can, to a lesser or greater degree, be expressed by individuals. Listening attentively to the communication within the baby boomer family is helpful in illuminating this facet of familial life under patriarchal capitalism today.

Chapter	**4**	THE ACCEPTANCE PROBLEM

Acceptance. For some baby boomers, that word says it all about the strain between themselves and their parents. A nod of approval, a show of interest, or a simple acknowledgment by parents that one's choices are respected is often as desired by the child at forty as it was at age four, yet often more difficult to get today than yesterday. Without parental approval, the baby boomers often find themselves feeling ambivalent toward their parents. Surrounding acceptance from parents is the issue of choice: choice of the baby boomer's career, lifestyle, spouse, and personal qualities.

"What's your gross income?"

The question "What's your gross income?" is not problematic for the baby boomers who have chosen conventional careers, but for those who have chosen to be artists, aerobic instructors, or herbalist. This question posed by their parents can drive a stake right through the heart of the family relationship. For example, Tom's father, a retired draftsman, cannot understand why his son is an artist instead of an engineer or something practical like the other kids in the family. For Tom, having a father who does not understand or respect his career choice is frustrating and the fountainhead of the animosity he feels toward his father. The questioning of Tom's career choice by his father gets to be an old tune after a while: "I resent my dad asking questions like 'What are you going to do?'"

"But you know, I don't hate his guts or anything," completed Tom. With tears in his eyes, Tom quietly spoke of the memory of his father lying in a hospital bed:

> When I saw my dad in the hospital with all those tubes and everything, heart-monitor, and not being able to talk and all that stuff. Well, anyway, it really bothered

me . . . . Sometimes now at night when I'm daydream-
ing, just thinking, I'll think of that image of him in the
hosptial and it bothers me.

The problem between Tom and his father is not lack of love but
the fact that Tom's father, to this day, has not acknowledged art as
a legitimate profession and, thus, his son as a full-fledged, responsible adult. It is as if Tom's father feels that in Tom becoming an
artist, he has done nothing with his life, even though he has
completed a terminal degree at the best college in his field, worked
very hard to become a master at his art, made a living at his artistic
profession for many years, and found great joy in being an artist.

Another baby boomer, Chris, spoke of a similar problem. Chris
is a world-renowned artist who last year accepted a position as a
professor of art at one of the top art schools in the United States. As
he put it, "Being an artist is as far away from their [his parents']
experience as possible." Chris's parents, who are divorced, wealthy,
and from Los Angeles, see him as a failure for what boils down to
his level of income. Success, in his parents' book, is measured by
dollars not by happiness:

> When they [his parents] ask at the end of the year how
> my year went, and I say I got into this museum and that
> museum, they say, "What was your gross income?"
> And it [his income] never measures up to their stan-
> dards; their gauge for how well someone is doing is his
> gross income and my whole gauge of whether you're a
> success is if you are happy or not.

Chris would like his parents to accept him for who he is and for
what he has accomplished in his life, so much so, that he does not
want them to die before they have given him their approval. As he
commented, "I wouldn't want my parents to die thinking that I was
a bum, I want them to recognize that I'm doing good and, consequently, they did good." But, for now, Chris's parents, especially his
mother, see little value in his work or lifestyle, and his mother
believes that someday he will "come around":

She thinks that something is going to click in my head,
and I'll turn my life around. She is convinced I've gone
down the wrong path, and that I'll somehow just come
to my senses. She just hasn't accepted that this is it!

Over the past few years, Chris has grown closer to his father as
a result of his father's willingness to let him lead his own life, even
though his father does not fully appreciate his profession. Chris's
mother has, as he put it, "never given in," but his father has
somewhat in that it means something to him that Chris is a professor
who is awarded grants and has work accepted in major museums
across the world. As time passes, Chris grows closer to his father and
further away from his mother.

One of the baby boomers already introduced in the study, Les,
fulfilled his father's dream by becoming an artist. His father, a kid
from the Bronx, had dropped out of high school to study art, but
times were hard during the Great Depression, so his education was
cut short. He went into window display to satisfy his artistic needs,
never to have the opportunity again to become a high-culture artist.
This is what Les remembers of the day he told his father of his plans
to become an artist: "I can remember my dad saying this with a
Jewish accent, 'Well, why you want to be an artist? How you going
to make a living?'"

Here, it was not the occupation that was questioned, but how the
young man was going to be able to survive as an artist in American
society. Les's father wished for Les "some wonderful faculty
teaching job or something." The wish came true, unfortunately, a
few months after the father's death. The "regular job," though, is still
good news to Les's mother who, finding herself at seventy-four
years of age living alone on a fixed income, is thankful she no longer
has to worry about her son struggling financially:

Well, my mom loves it that I have a job now instead of
a free-lance potter. But, what's the bottom line there is
the concern that I don't have to struggle . . . When you
work at a "regular job" as I do now, you have health
insurance . . . if you're on your own, as artists are, health
insurance is out of their reach, they fall behind the
cracks, fall through the cracks. And, also the money

isn't regular. So, I think my mom is thinking, "Oh, he has a steady job, so he can get some of the things he wants." Although, when I was selling pots, I was doing all right.

Along with the bottom dollar is the color, figuratively speaking, of the baby boomer's collar. Dan, the sign painter, says his parents are disappointed in him for having chosen a blue-collar profession instead of a white-collar one:

> It's like I did not become the person they wanted, and that really hurt my dad more than anybody . . . . Evidently, I'm suppose to go from his [dad's] blue-collar to a white-collar job. And I just didn't cut that.

When Dan, Les, Chris, and Tom are asked "What's your gross income?" by their parents, they are being confronted with the whole societal ball of wax. The question exemplifies what is important in this society: money and social rank. Though the question is often asked by parents out of genuine love and concern for the welfare of their adult children, it represents societal values, conventions, and class differentials that are at the core of American society. It presents this choice to the baby boomers: Conform and win parental approval, or take the risk of nonconformity at the cost of losing love and respect from your parents. What is being generated is the feeling of ambivalence. The parental pressure experienced by the baby boomers to pursue jobs that "pay well" or are "practical" or are "white collar" is, in actuality, part of the larger authoritarian structure that attempts to force individuals to not only succeed monetarially, to not only conform to the social order, but to cherish the class structure as well.

"This is not what we expected!"

The "This is not what we expected!" theme song of the parents carries over into many facets of the baby boomers' lives, including their career goals, lifestyles, and marriage partners, and this can be a real sore spot in the intergenerational relationship. For instance, Cathy, the editor, finds herself being a different person from the individual her parents had expected. What her parents wanted for her was to be a "happy homemaker" whose whole identity was wrapped up in her family. Instead, Cathy is a person who needs and wants more than her family to feel she is living a "full life." She enjoys her career, the arts, and literature, none of which her parents have ever appreciated. At this point in her life, Cathy would like to go back to college and complete a Ph.D., another ambition her parents think is ludicrous. Her parents' seemingly total disregard for what she wants from life has resulted in Cathy's feeling emotionally distant from her parents, though bonded.

Patricia, who owns and operates an alternative aerobics fitness center has, over the years, experienced marked disapproval from her mother in trying to develop a life of her own. For instance, when Patricia was fresh out of college and living near her parents, her mother was very upset with her for living a life separate from the family:

> My experience, particularly from my mother, being . . . [that she was] not very supportive of me as a separate unit from the family . . . . When I bought a house of my own, a great deal of anger and nastiness that I experienced from my mother, in particular, which I identify as being a frustration with my leaving the nest, my being separate. And there were constant expectations of me to be at their house to do things for them, to do things with them even though I was in my twenties. And, I was very resistant and as a result, I experienced a great deal of anger from my mother.

Today, the expectations Patricia has for herself are still different from those her mother, now widowed, has for her. Patricia has chosen to live across the country from her family, to operate her own aerobics business, and to have an alternative lifestyle, in spite of her mother's wishing she would live close to her, have a "real job," and live as "normal people" do. Not surprisingly, Patricia said, "I don't feel especially close to my parents, to my mother, nor do I feel especially distant, I feel rather neutral." Yet Patricia cares enough about her mother to write her a letter about every two weeks, send her gifts for holidays and birthdays, and call her as often as she can afford to do so.

A small-business manager in upstate New York named Cheri told me that it took a long time for her parents to accept her husband,

and that this is a source for ill feelings even today. Her parents (her mother a director of archives at the university library, her father a retired college professor and now owner of the small business) had expected that she would leave her small, college town and move on to "go for the stars." As it turned out, Cheri stayed in town, married a local boy, had kids, settled into a routine life just around the corner from where her parents live, and became co-owner of her father's business. Recognition for what Cheri has accomplished and how far she has gone in her life has been less forthcoming from her father than from her mother:

> They [her parents] were hoping great things for me . . .
> You hear so many things like "go for the stars," but I
> think Mom anyway appreciates how far I've gone and
> what I've done. I think Pop does but he has a hard time
> admitting it . . . . He doesn't give much . . . . recognition
> to what I'm doing.

In Cheri's case, the subject of parental expectations has been compounded by the fact the her parents are not only her parents but also her employers, who control her income. Parental expectations overlap between the personal and the business, which at times makes for a tough situation for Cheri, and one that is heightened when Cheri cannot converse with her parents, a common occurrence, according to her.

Still, Cheri feels close to her parents and is proud of them. She has always been her father's "shadow," always following him around, and she was there to support him and her mother when her father was being treated for cancer, an experience that Cheri says prepared her for taking care of her folks later on, if need be.

In another case, the problem was that the man's mother had difficulty "letting go" of him, mainly because she did not like her son's wife. As described by Robert, "She [his mother] was trying to keep track of me a lot when I was first married . . . . I don't think to be nosy, but . . . my first wife and her didn't get a long." After the marriage ended in divorce, all was fine between mother and son. And when Robert remarried, the problem did not arise, so the son is sure it had to do with the chemistry between his mother and his first wife. Still, the episode has not been forgotten, and is one that is remembered for causing "many, many problems."

In the stories mentioned so far, the parents at some point in time were accepting of their children's spouses. Sometimes, the parents never reach even neutral ground concerning their children's partners. Jill made this comment about her mother: "And when it comes to her daughters, there are no men that are good enough for any of us; so, she has a hard time accepting anyone in our lives." Jill's mother, herself twice divorced and now widowed, would prefer that her daughters be independent of men, which she was not and now regrets. Her attitude is that her daughters will have better lives (i.e., more stable and financially secure lives) without the men.

That many of the baby boomers' parents think they have the right to pressure their adult children into conformity is evident in their "This is not what we expected!" reaction. The reaction creates tension between the generations because it is an exercise of parental authority to force the baby boomers to blend into their parents' social milieu. When the offspring resist the wishes of their parents, they again suffer ambivalence. Parents like Cathy's, who want their daughters to be homemakers; mothers like Patricia's, who do not want their daughters to live independent of the family; professional couples like Cheri's parents, who want their children to "go for the stars"; and the many mothers like Robert's and Jill's, who disapprove of the children's spouses—all have in common a wish for their children to be their little shadows, by desiring what they desire and by fulfilling the needs that they need to have fulfilled. The parental reactions get down to authority and dominance, the same dynamics that exist outside the family in American society. From the American family to American society, the organization is protected because the underlings have internalized what the authority figures expect of them, and though the individuals may challenge some expectations, they will not discredit the right of the authority. The shadows have been cast.

"Do you approve, Mom and Dad?"

Some baby boomers, especially women, find themselves in their everyday lives wondering about or even doing things that they know would meet with their parents' approval. For example, a nurse in Portland said, "I remember when I was younger and living at home that I did try to do things that would give me my parents' approval, and, as an adult now, I also like to do those kinds of things that make my parents happy." A medical technologist living in Buffalo said she associates completing her college degree with showing her parents that she is a responsible person. At the other side of New York State, a mother of two boys in Albany explained to me that the reason she got a slow start on her professional career was because she stayed home for several years after her children were born mainly because she knew it would please her parents. Another mother of two boys who is a clerk living in the Southern Tier of New York admitted that she has tried to rear her children in such a way as to get her parents' approval.

When Maria, a New England resident whose mother is a homemaker and father a retired ocean tanker navigator, thought about seeking her parents' approval, this is what came to her mind:

> When I think of approval now, I think in the back of my mind, it's funny, I still do. A lot of times, even when I'm picking out furniture, and my mother and I have very different tastes, I think, "I bet my mother wouldn't like that," or if I have some decisions to do about something, "This isn't what she'd pick." And than I begin to feel a little bit of guilt in maybe picking something that she would not have picked or making a decision she would not have made.

From picking out furniture to making decisions, the concern to please her mother remains at the forefront of Maria's consciousness. Maria finished her thought by saying that what her mother would approve of is still sort of the "standard for what is really the right thing to do or the right decision to make." Yet Maria is a forty-four-year-old wife, mother, and experienced medical researcher. Later in the interview, when Maria responded to whether she shared the same values as her parents, she reflected on how very difficult it is for her to relax, for her impulse is to feel guilty if she is not busy doing something constructive. Maria's reaction stems from the strong work ethic embedded in her mind by her parents:

> I guess basically we do [share the same values], but my parents have this extremely strong . . . work ethic. There's nothing in the world as good as to work, work,

work at whatever you're doing . . . . Taking time for fun
or just relaxation or whatever . . . is looked down upon
. . . Just sitting down to relax is pretty much a "no-no."
I feel I have to get so much accomplished . . . but I also
feel that you spend [time] relaxing with your children,
vacations, just sitting around talking, staying home
watching television, going to a movie . . . . And I know
this is something my parents would feel like you're
wasting your time, you shouldn't be doing that . . . . And
sometimes it's hard for me, I feel guilty doing things I
know that they would not necessarily approve of.

A homemaker living in Connecticut whose name is Elizabeth
and whose standard of living is "very close to that of my friends who
came from families that were quite well off financially, very well off
financially" also found herself striving to please her parents
throughout her childhood, adolescence, and early adulthood years.
Today, she maintains a comfortable lifestyle with her husband, a
physician. Elizabeth said that the need to please her mother has been
the "driving force" in her life, though the need is not as pronounced
today as it once was:

But this was something that was a driving force [in my
life], the need to please my mother . . . . I don't make the
desire to please my mother a central issue in my life now
as an adult. Although I will go out of my way to have
things be the way she would like for them to be in the
house or serve something she would like to eat or make
a fuss about something she would like a fuss made about
when they [her parents] do come to visit me.

Another woman, Ellen, ended up getting married at age thirty-
six in spite of her distaste for the institution of marriage. She and her
companion of several years wanted to have a child and knew that
having a child out of wedlock would test their parents' level of
acceptance to the limit:

I knew it would be very hard for my parents to accept a
child that was born out of wedlock even after many
years of living with the same man. And [the man] also

felt it would be much easier for his parents. So we got married for our parents to approve of this child which we'll have sometime in the future. I think that's a pretty big issue, because I still sometimes wish I weren't married just because I don't have a lot of respect for the institution of marriage.

The way a part-time librarian in Albany named Janice said she keeps from seeking her parents' approval as much as she did as a child is by flat-out refusing to tell them anything they would not approve of, or at least waiting until much later in time to bring up what is now safely history. In her words: "If I do something that I know they don't approve of, then I usually don't tell them or I'll wait a long time before I tell them." A similar stratgey was employed by Maria who suggested that she has her parents' support because she has yet to inform them of anything that would upset them:

I guess I've really never done anything that they wouldn't be supportive of. I never wanted to run away to Australia, live on the streets somewhere or something like that. I haven't done anything major that they wouldn't accept. So, basically, whatever I wanted they would help monetarially and emotionally as much as they were able to.

The willingness of the baby boomers to show deference to parental authority is characterized in their conscious efforts to please their parents. Particular aspects of the baby boomers' desire to please their parents stem from the structure of the privatized American family. The need to please parents was all-important during the baby boomers' preschool years when their parents were their exclusive role models and sources of love and praise on a daily basis. And because child rearing was left almost entirely to mothers, the baby boomers' mothers, in the seriousness of their assignment, were rigid, threatening withdrawal of love if their children misbehaved and, as products of their time, supporting traditional sex roles. As a consequence, the baby boomers grew up with experiences of ambivalence and sex-role differentiation.

The experiences have resulted in adult children, especially daughters, who are keenly aware of what is pleasing to their parents, especially their mothers, and the consequences if their parents are not pleased. Adult daughters, more than adult sons, have this awareness because of the traditional sex-role expectation that daughters be "proper," "lady-like." And mothers, more than fathers, because children spent more time with their mothers, whose personhood was packaged in "motherhood," came to learn more of their expectations and reactions. This explains why adult daughters like Maria and Elizabeth are still asking the question, "Do you approve, Mom?" The question helps maintain the adult child's conformity; it reinforces parental authority, offspring inferiority, and, overall, a tradition of domination from within the individual that is needed to keep the abiding self-motivation high in an advanced capitalist patriarchal society.

It is clear from the preceding interviews that the baby boomers take very much to heart the approval of their parents. The baby boomers want and need their parents to accept them for who and what they are, so much so in fact that some walk around tormented because they are pursuing a passion their parents mock, while others forego certain joys in life or withhold certain truths about themselves from their parents. Acceptance breeds ambivalence and conformity to the current social order; when the baby boomers are confronted with it, they are confronted with all that is precious and sacred to the American way of life.

Given the nature of acceptance (from parent to child) in the intergenerational relationship, I regard it as the key component of the emotional context of the adult child, the component that both perpetuates ambivalent feelings toward the parents and reinforces social conformity. The emotional burden is still between personal gratification and parental love, only now that the pleasures go beyond bodily functions to that of the heart and mind of the adult child. The reason the burden seems inescapable to the baby boomers is obviously not because of the confines of the home, as in childhood, but because the confines are embedded so deeply in the adult child's soul and are sustained by the impersonal and dehumanizing nature of an everyday world where love and care are so hard to find.

Parental authority is still terrifying for the baby boomers because they do not want to hate, or be hated by, persons they love and who love them. They know that their parents are not going to change and that if they, the offspring, refuse to change, then they must face the torment of threats from their parents. Such threats may include being thought of as an "irresponsible husband" or a "bum" or a "bad mother" or a "lazy person" or a "disrespectful child," and on and on. The adult children face a situation where anger cannot be directed against their parents for fear of rejection, so it is internalized against themselves, resulting in feelings of guilt, doubts of self-worth, dissatisfaction with their situation, not to mention puzzlement and bewilderment. Some chuckle, some cry over their inability to break away from the stronghold of their parents. Whether the baby boomers like it or not, they are forced by their parents to confront the social order as it exists.

More concretely, the emotional structure of the older family's relations helps generate attitudes of respectability, which are absolutely essential for upholding the status quo. Fear of parental rejection among adult children fosters conformity and autonomy: conformity in the sense that adult children show deference to parental authority, autonomy in the sense that adult children see themselves as independent whenever they consciously choose personal pleasure over parental approval. The combination is just what the larger social organization of society needs: individuals enmeshed in the authority structure who still feel independent of it. In this way, individuals continue to be ignorant of the forces of domination looming over them.

THE PARENTAL-CONTROL PROBLEM

Chapter **5**

Another factor identified by the baby boomers that can be associated with the tension between them and their parents is the sum of attempts by their parents to control their lives from childhood onward. Parents who actively seek to control their adult children's lives have not relinquished their position of authority over their children. They still seek to have a direct influence on their children by letting their offspring know what they approve or disapprove of, or by trying to meddle in their children's' affairs, or by manipulating funds that affect their children's current or future condition. Whatever the particular circumstance may be, the outcome is the same: The baby boomers feel considerable animosity toward their parents.

"Because I'm your mother!"

Many of the baby boomers complained of mothers who were overbearing, who felt they had a right to force their will on them. For example, consider what happened between Elizabeth and her parents:

> During my childhood, my mother tended to be a very controlling person. I didn't question what she told me to do . . . in the time I was in college, and the time right after and early in my marriage, I did feel that my mother felt that she could control me. That her opinions were the only opinions that were tolerated and that I couldn't know too much that she knew everything and knew the right way to do things. I have to admit that probably she had too profound an effect on my decision making in those years prior to the time that I became depressed.

A big part of the reason Elizabeth became depressed is reflected in the way her mother treated her as a child:

> I can remember her finding fault with me frequently whenever we went somewhere, things I had said were dumb, or things I did were dumb. I didn't really hear about the wonderful things I did . . . . I did not feel very confident of myself, and I tended to be self-conscious. My mother frequently would tell me that I could be better at this or better at that. I felt that I wasn't pretty enough, that I wasn't thin enough, that I wasn't smart enough, that I wasn't aggressive enough. I only knew what I wasn't enough of and not what I was adequate at.

Although Elizabeth resented the criticism from her mother, she prided herself on being a "perfect child":

> I didn't question what she [her mother] told me to do. I obeyed and did whatever I was told to do, and I'm described by my parents as the "perfect girl." That I was such a good girl, they never had to worry about me and I never sneaked around and misbehaved. I, from what they say, was the epitome of good behavior.

The toll for seeking perfection was a depressed young woman who eventually wound up in counseling. After four months of counseling, Elizabeth emerged as a much less depressed and a much more "assertive and self-directed" individual, which created stress between her and her mother: "My mother still wanted to control me, and I was not receptive to that, and it was hard for her to accept." During this period, the relationship between Elizabeth and her mother was strained; it began to improve over time, and today Elizabeth rates the relationship as "basically quite good."

The reflections noted by Elizabeth enliven the impression that the presence of parental control plagues the intergenerational relationship. Parental control is about domination, the disease of capitalist patriarchal society. It epitomizes a mentality stuck on hierarchical stackings. The thinking in a capitalist patriarchal society is vertical not horizontal; thoughts are geared toward social rankings

(Gray 1982). The ranking of individuals in organizations, including the family, is based on power, a power restricted to who is on top, be it teacher, boss, police officer, judge—or husband, or parent. In the family, the traditional ranking puts father on top, then mother, and then their children by age and sex.

The rejoinder "Because I'm your mother!" is one example of vertical thinking. These few words tell much about the domination of women and children in our society. They tell how mothers, relegated by their sex to subordinate positions in the society, exert what little power they have over their offspring. The mothers are, of course, threatened when their adult children break loose from their authority. After all, what authority is left to most older women in this society? What do most of them truly control beyond such superficials as the color of their hair, the brand of soap they use, and the times they should send off the mail or go to bed. Also, the mothers are encumbered with the notion that the perfect child (i.e., the child who has perfectly conformed to the requirements of the society) is a reflection of the perfect mother. The loss of power coupled with the burden of being "perfect mothers" add up in many cases to mothers anxiously attempting to wield what little power they have over their adult children.

This puts Elizabeth and some other baby boomers in a peculiar position. On the one hand, the adult children have been brought up to cherish their independence and to exercise it as adults; on the other hand, they have been raised to be, as dependents, respectful of their parents. When mothers solicit deference from their adult children, in essence they are forcing their children to choose between individual freedom and maternal affection. The dilemma is another example of the new emotional structure where adult children face the ambivalent pulls between personal satisfaction and parental love.

"We were just wondering . . ."

Attempts by parents to control their offspring's lives come in a variety of packages, one of which has to do with trying to become too involved in their children's personal affairs. There is a point at which parents overstep the bounds of their parental authority, and when this happens, the general reaction from the baby boomers is one of exasperation. For example, Anna, a town clerk living in the Northeast, said that she does not feel close to her parents because "they get overinvolved . . . sometimes they want to know more than I think they should know." This is what upsets Anna:

> It's . . . aggravating . . . when they're trying to pry something out of me, like maybe there's a problem between my husband and [me] or something like that, they just can't take "No!" for an answer . . . . They feel they have to know, and that bothers me . . . I feel they're my parents, but they don't need to know everything . . . some things aren't any of their business. I don't think they can accept that real well.

The problem of parents wanting to know all the details of their adult child's life has turned into a nightmare for Sharon, a medical technologist, who charges that her parents use the personal information as source material for trying to convert her to their religious ways. Never mind that Sharon is thirty-three years old and has her own religious beliefs. Recently, Sharon's mother and stepfather drove to Buffalo from Kansas, unannounced, to take her back to Kansas, because they thought she was living an immoral life and wanted to "save" her. When she made a light joke of the whole affair in an effort to downplay the gravity of it, her parents turned their car around that same afternoon and drove back to Kansas. That is the last time Sharon saw her parents.

"My mother is a constant pest!" complained Chris, the glass sculptor. His well-to-do mother is a "pest" because when she calls twice a week and comes to visit twice a year, she wants to know when her son plans to change his lifestyle and get back "in line."

While visiting, she never fails to have something to say about the latest "twist on the will" or to seize the opportunity to take Chris's wife off to the side and ask, "Why don't you move back to the city?" The "city" representing material wealth and creature comforts. Chris' mother still asks him, "Do you need socks? underwear? furniture?" If he does, she gets them for him as soon as possible and ships them by rapid carrier, along with items for his wife and baby. Yes the pestiness is an outgrowth of concern, but it is also, according to Chris, part of his mother's desire to make the statement to him that he cannot provide for his family, though he can, and the statement that she is still a major influence in his life.

The parents of Anna, Sharon, and Chris are trying to exert influence in their children's lives, though their efforts have been checked by the baby boomers. Why do parents bother to interfere in their adult children's personal business? Because the ability of parents to intrude successfully into their adult children's lives is a sign to all, including the parents, that their parental authority perseveres. This pattern is seen no less often outside the home where, in a society that thrives on hierarchical structures, the dominant members need to have their authority reinforced from time to time. Reinforcement reassures the oppressors that the oppressed are not going to seek emancipation. Thus reinforcement not only comforts the insecurities of the authority figures but also sustains the established order of society. Be it in the home or outside the home, the authoritarian structure is bent on domination in a form that does not appear to be what it is. One way individuals are blinded to the forces that dominate them is through the reinforcement of authority in the home where it seems rooted in a biological right. Constant subjection to reinforcement in the private realm accustoms the children to the reinforcement to come in the public realm. When individuals finally confront a larger authoritarian structure, it seems familiar to them and is regarded as a natural arrangement.

"We know what's best for you, Sweetheart!"

The sentiment that parents know what is best for their adult children is frequently encountered by the baby boomers, and it is a constant source of strife between the generations. Everything from being told how to speak properly to when it is appropriate to marry comes across loud and clear to the baby boomers. For example, a man who has a college degree, served ten years in Africa as a conscientious objector and social worker, and now writes a monthly newsletter for an environmental group, says his mother "is a real stickler for grammar and language, and if you mispronounce a word . . . you're persona non grata." Another baby boomer begrudgingly hears out her mother on how she and her siblings should behave. In yet another case, an established artist impatiently listens to her mother telling her to draw "something more refined." And one woman finds that her parents, who are also her employer, decide on an "appropriate amount" for her annual income.

Jane, a homemaker who is working on a master's degree in art education at a private college in upstate New York, located about 250 miles from where her parents live, told me that she would not want to live near her parents:

> I see what my brother and sister have to endure ....Mom has always been overpowering, always very domineering, and she to this day finds terrible fault with my brother rearing his children ....Poor [sister and brother] living so nearby, [mom] wants their children to have those same perfect lives that she didn't have and that she wanted us to be so perfect and now obviously she wants her grandchildren to be that way, that's tough for the kids.

Several baby boomers talked about how their parents had been heavy-handed in matters about their college education, and how, over the years, this has affected their lives and their relationships with their parents. Laurie, a forty-year-old women whose father is a retired bureaucrat in Albany, New York, and whose mother has always been a homemaker, accounted for her ill feelings toward her parents by the fact that when she was ready to go to college, her parents gave her an ultimatum: Go to college in Albany or do not go at all. The college of her choice was outside Albany, and so Laurie never made it to college and today is employed in a clerical position.

The ill feelings are real, but so are the loving feelings between Laurie and her parents, a fact revealed when Laurie explained why she felt close to her parents:

> Well, because they [her parents] have always wanted to be involved in my life and what I'm doing. I feel ... they love me and I love them. They care. They care about what happens to us.

Along the same line, Cynthia, a single woman working as a psychiatric counselor in Oregon, lost all financial support for her college education from her parents, both mathematicians at the college level in California, because she would not stop being a "radical" and would not quit the college of her choice in order to move back home, as her parents demanded:

> When I was in college, I went to a fairly radical college in the '70s, and came home espousing a variety of ideas with which my mother in particular, but my father as well, were not very pleased . . . . In my sophomore year my mother decided to withdraw all parental support from me unless I agreed to come home and live at home and toe the line . . . . I would not bend to their will.

Cynthia ended up quitting college and going to work for a couple of years. After she saved the money for her education, she went back to her chosen college and finished her degree; she now works at a psychiatric crisis center in Oregon. Her parents did not attend her graduation, nor did they ever acknowledge it beyond a, "Glad you finally finished school." Cynthia was hurt by her parents' indifference toward her college endeavors. The wound is still healing some fourteen years later.

Michael ended up having to explain to his father, a retired academician, why, after completing his master's degree, he did not go on for his Ph.D. (he did not need a Ph.D. for the position he desired, nor did he value education as "the be-all and end-all"). The expectation that Michael would complete a Ph.D. was ground into him at an early age:

> I can remember from my very earliest teen years my father talking to various people and it always had to do with education: "Get that bachelor's degree! Get that master's degree! Get that Ph.D.!" and just harassed my brother who stopped about six hours short from a master's. I had a very clear sense that that was important to them [his parents].

As an adult, Michael has distanced himself from his parents' influence by not asking them for their opinion, though he knows that "that [is] something they would probably value a lot."

Breaking tradition has its price, as one thirty-five-year-old librarian living outside Albany contests. The affinity between her and her parents was damaged many years ago when her parents refused to attend her wedding because of their strong disapproval over her having lived with her fiance for a year. And when her parents attended the wedding of her sister, the baby boomer's heart "cracked like ice."

The lives of Michael, Cynthia, Laurie, Jane, and other baby boomers have continued within an authoritarian structure. For the inferior, life within an authoritarian structure has few choices except the ones offered by superiors. Until individuals are financially independent, they are placed in the lowly position of having to abide by the prerogatives of the money holders. This financial circumstance underlies the parents' affirmation that they know what is best for their children. The parents, over the years, present their children with various choices that are basically a collection of societal values.

What is unique to the postbourgeois structure is that once the children become adults, they are financially independent of their parents and immersed in a world where mass media and other societal sources provide them with an array of possibilities. But there is still this one problem: Parents do not want to relinquish their authority over their adult children. They still want to prescribe the confines of their children's choices, in part because in the larger scheme of things they have so little to control and in part because the status of their adult children is regarded as a reflection of their own respectability. Again, the adult children combat ambivalence.

"This is good news!"

Not all news is bad news to parents. Some news is good news. The "good news" is news that the baby boomers are doing something perfectly conventional—buying a house, settling into a job, getting married, having children—and are doing it in an orthodox fashion. Take, as an example, Dan from Portland, Oregon. He explained that while he does not actively seek his parents' approval, he is aware that more of the things he is doing now please them, and these are the things he chooses to share with his parents:

> I think more of the things I'm feeling now are estab-
> lished sort of things: owning a house, living with a
> Jewish girl type of thing. And those are more appropriate
> to their [his parents'] values, so, I think they are, they're
> more approving. There are still some things that I'm
> doing that they would not approve of, but those are
> things that they don't know about . . . . You don't tell
> your parents everything.

"My mother was happy that my husband and I finally married, and then when we gave her two grandsons and one granddaughter, she was in heaven!" So says a Kansas woman who works part-time as a bank teller. A schoolteacher who moved to Connecticut, some distance from the state of Washington where his parents reside, said that his moving to Connecticut came as a "shock" to his parents, "but they were glad to see that maybe I was going to get married." Similarly, a graduate student said his parents were better able to handle his move from the Midwest to the East Coast because he and his wife of nearly ten years, after "settling in" at their new residence, had a baby, something his parents had been wanting to see happen for many years.

Following convention is paramount to respectability. Getting married, having kids, buying a house, succeeding professionally are the facets of convention most pleasing to the parents of baby boomers. While alternative lifestyles—living together or living in a homosexual household, choosing not to have children or having children out of wedlock, sharing a residence with others, or opting for a career outside the mainstream—are often reproved by the parents, the orthodox is celebrated. Baby boomers now in their thirties and forties heed, to a degree, the words spoken by their parents. Parental control lives on. Parental control instills respectability in the baby boomers; it also perpetuates ambivalence because it forces children to choose between parental love and a desired lifestyle.

Parental control is part and parcel of domination in the American family drama. It commits age and sex discrimination to the realm of tradition, and it ensures that youngsters are prepared for the more crushing authoritarian structures outside the family world. The master lesson it sends is that individualism should not exceed tradition. That is, individualism is about being part of the system, not about being part of challenging it. This is what we have come to know as respectability. Plainly, parental control is a major component of domination in the United States that helps protect the status quo.

Chapter	**6**	TRADITIONAL FAMILY DYNAMICS

Traditional family dynamics were spotlighted by many of the baby boomers as a major grievance regarding their intergenerational relationships. The "aloof" father and the "milktoast" mother were mentioned in particular. The general complaint voiced by the baby boomers was about how traditional sex roles and their accompanying expectations have interfered with the quality of the relationship between themselves and their parents.

"We're just one big happy family!"

The family world of the baby boomers was steeped in traditional sex roles. Father went to work each day, mother stayed home, and the children caught the brunt of the role demands of their parents, making for a less than wonderful and loving household. Many baby boomers look back on their childhoods and have regrets about what was and what could have been, and how all this has affected their adult child/parent relationships. One of regret is that fathers were seldom home, and when they were around, they failed to take the time to do things with the baby boomers or to show them that they loved and cared for them. As Dan remarked:

> I feel close to my mom, a lot closer than my dad. He always kept a distance from us, and he felt that his best parenting could be done by giving us a secure financial base. Which is a horse-shit rationalization, because [my brother] and I really feel like we have not spent time with our father when we would have really liked to. He rarely played with us. I don't know, his role model must have really been a bad one. His dad was pretty much the same as him.

Grandfathers, as well as fathers, were described as poor role models by Elizabeth. In responding to why she has always felt close to her parents, Elizabeth turned to an aspect of her family history in which we can note her relational thinking:

> I think I've always felt close to my parents. In my childhood . . . my father was always working or busy doing something . . . . So, therefore, I spent most of my time with my mother. When my father was growing up as a youngster, his dad was never home, he worked constantly. And he would come home essentially for meals and to go to bed. And he really had nothing to do with the rearing of the children, that was left solely up to my grandmother, his mother. In my mother's case, somewhat the same thing though my grandfather was home more often . . . he tended to be more disinterested and more selfish with his time, and my mother was not that close to her father when she grew up.

Elizabeth went on to explain that although she did not see much of her father when she was growing up, she nonetheless has always felt attached to him, mainly because he had a good sense of humor and was willing to buy her whatever she wanted:

> I always remember him [her father] as being very kind with a wonderful sense of humor and willing to do anything you'd like for you. Whatever I wanted in terms of material things he wanted me to have. There were never any questions, I could have twenty pairs of shoes and want another pair of shoes and say, "Dad, I want to get another pair of shoes," and that would be fine . . . . I had a car in high school, a car that was quite an expensive sports car, and I always had many beautiful clothes. I always had many material things.

What is interesting about Dan's and Elizabeth's comments is the "role model factor" and the emphasis on "the material basis of life," which touch on both the ideological socialization process and the role assignments steming from the separation between work and home. The roles their fathers took on were the ones passed down to them by *their* fathers, the ones deemed appropriate in a society where men are expected to be self-reliant providers and women nurturers, interconnected with others. Both Dan and Elizabeth are bonded to their fathers, but clearly desire a more interactive relationship with them.

The same is true for David, a potter living in upstate New York. He said that the "biggest" reason he has ill feelings toward his father is his father's "separateness from the children in things that they did in their personal lives, that he didn't participate, well, very little as far as like taking us to school or playing games with us or anything of this, my mother did that." The "separateness from the children" has carried over to include the grandchildren, something that David said bothered him "a lot." David finished his thoughts by detailing how he is making a conscious effort not to follow his father's example. One difference is that he works at home, which makes it easier for him to be physically near his children. Also, when he has finished his work for the day, David often engages his children in activities with him—playing catch, preparing dinner, or just talking—all of which help give the "father model" a new image.

"Because he was cruel . . . things that he could control . . . he took advantage of . . . . I thought he was overbearing toward us kids, but weak in other respects," was the answer given by Joe, a technician in upstate New York, as to why he did not feel close to his father, a retired factory worker. The father's cruelty, combined with his poor "financial head," added up to a life of hardship for Joe, his siblings, and his mother. Consequently, Joe said that he "probably wouldn't feel anything" if his father died, but should he lose his mother, he would feel "a deep loss."

The situation Joe found himself in while growing up is a classic example of what Marx and Engels called "father-right." Father-right refers to the unchecked authority of the father under capitalism, which emerged with the rise of the state. Joe's father faced an authoritarian structure in the factory, submission forced on him by the money holders; at home, he reigned over his wife and children for the same reasons his superiors had power over him. Given the authoritarian structure of the work world, home was the only place where Joe's father could have control over something—a sorry situation for Joe, his siblings, and his mother which today plagues the intergenerational relationship between Joe and his aging father.

Suzanne, who grew up in Tennessee, offered the following in clarification of her feelings toward her "typical southern father" when he was living: "I think I was angry with my father in that I didn't feel that he showed enough . . . that he loved me, I wish he had more." Earlier in the interview, Suzanne, now settled in the Southern Tier of New York with her husband, daughter, and son, interpreted "typical southern father" in its relevance to her past life and to how she has redefined relations in her own home:

> The southern father, possibly not anymore, but in the
> past was king of the house. And you waited on the father,
> you poured his iced tea or whatever he needed . . . [you]
> definitely showed deference. And even for my brothers,
> I was expected to get up and pour tea for them, to wait
> on them. Their comforts when they were in the home
> were high priority. Of course, I rebelled from all of that,
> all of it, completely. I'm very much independent from
> all of that now. My life is just as important as everyone
> else's.

From what Suzanne said, her family was a site for "exploitation exchanges of services," as Fraser has claimed families usually are under capitalism. Being female in a patriarchical setting directly affected Suzanne's relations with other family members. The servant like role she was placed in demeaned her worth as a human being while elevating the males in her family, spelling out a separation between the sexes that would limit displays of affection from father to daughter. In her family of orientation, Suzanne would always be the inferior and her father the unemotional superior.

Traditional fathers, in general, were rational, insensitive beings who ruled over, more than they interacted with, their children. They had little patience with their offspring, perhaps because in spending so little time with them, they were ignorant about the abilities and personalities of their youngsters. Regardless, the critical factor is the damage done to the intergenerational relationship as the result of the behavior of traditional fathers. The following quote by Maria targets the damage done in her case and some of the specifics behind it:

> Since my father was not there a great deal of the time,
> I was not particularly close to him. Also, when he came
> home, there was nothing that I could do that would

please him. Whatever I did there was something the matter with it and he would end up getting furious, yelling at me . . . . It was always traumatic whether it was going bowling when I was six years old, having the wrong form or something, or not holding the board the right way when he was sawing it.

Not only were traditional fathers impatient and difficult to please, they were also disciplinarians in the family, which added to the harshness of the interactions, as Meredith explained about her father, who was an engineer in the Deep South:

> I have never felt close to my father. My father is very emotionally withdrawn . . . . He was the disciplinarian in the family, I was the oldest kid, I caught a lot of the flack. He blamed me for a lot of things I never felt was fair . . . . As an adult, my father and I don't talk a whole lot. I feel pretty estranged from him.

In scenarios where the fathers were absent from the home, the setting was different but not the characters (except in one case where the baby boomer, a black woman who grew up in Alabama, did not know her father and was raised by her aunt). There were still fathers who remained at an emotional arms' length from their children, as Joyce, the daughter of an attorney in Oregon, affirmed:

> My relationship with my father was never real close . . . . He wasn't exactly cruel, but if you did something wrong, he always would scold you for it. It made me feel uncomfortable. After Mom and Dad got divorced, he used to see us every week. He'd take us places, trying to be nice in his own way, but we never developed any close relationship. And now that he's older, he doesn't remember what went on. He thinks he was a perfect dad.

Another daughter of a divorce, Diane, a medical technologist from Buffalo, had this to say about her father (now retired from his own business, the father vacations in Florida over the winter months):

> I resent my father because I think he probably could
> have been more helpful in my life. He has the finances
> to help me out a little bit more. He was always saying,
> "You don't get anything without working for it" and
> really forced me to accept that point . . . . But when
> you're only ten or eleven, it's a hard lesson to learn. I
> think he was excessive. I think there were times he could
> have been there for me when I was growing up, but he
> wasn't.

Jill, the daughter in a different divorce that took place before she
was born, has more sympathy for her father, an airline pilot back
then, even though he was not a "perfect dad":

> My daddy was quite the good-lookin', do-whatever-he-
> wanted type of man and sure had his share of ladies. I
> think my father's heart was in the right direction whether
> he expressed it or not. And I know that he loved us, even
> though he didn't actually help support us like he should
> of. He wasn't there to offer the support and help that we
> needed during our lives . . . . I have had ill feelings
> toward Father for not doing some of those things, not
> being there, not giving me the moral support . . . of what
> I thought it meant to be a daughter . . . . [But] I love my
> father . . . and always will.

The love loss was much more pronounced with Angie, whose
father, a factory supervisor in a small town in Ohio, virtually
abandoned his young family, being more interested in fast cars,
drink, and women than the well-being of his wife and children.
Throughout Angie's upbringing, the family relied on handouts from
other family members, friends, and neighbors for its basic needs.
Angie, now an artist, feels her relationship with her father was a false
one in that there were times when, under the prompting of her
mother, she would ask her father to buy her something she desper-
ately needed. "In that way, I felt I had a false relationship with my
father, because I knew that if I was going to get schoolbooks or
shoes, I would have to talk him into buying them for me."

Angie concluded her interview with the following account of the
problem behind the ill feelings she has toward her mother:

I think she [her mother] would have done better [han-
dling the divorce, raising the children as a single parent]
if she'd been born in another age where, maybe, see,
she's so sensitive to what the expectation for the female
role is, that I'm sure that that was most of the problem
with her trying to find work, trying to get out of a
marriage that didn't work, all the sort of social pressure
in a small town that worked against her. She has a very
conventional sense of how things ought to be, and I
think that worked against her.

Under capitalist patriarchy, traditional fathers are breadwinners.
When they live up to this expectation and are responsive and jovial
toward their children during the rare moments they spend with them,
the filial bond is strengthened, as in the case of Elizabeth. When the
expectation is met without the emotional component intact (as
Maria, Meredith, and Joyce have shown), the bond, although there,
is weakened. When the expectation is not met, the outcome is like
that of Joe, Diane, Angie, and Jill; the children think less of their
fathers, though they might make excuses for them, as did Jill.
Coupled with emotional estrangement (as with Joe, Diane, and
Angie), the end result can be children feeling indifferent toward their
fathers.

Their fathers' buying things sometimes was a good indicator of
the terms of the intergenerational relationship, creating disillu-
sionment on the part of baby boomers toward their parents, as in a
few of the cases mentioned above. Moreover, the material role of the
father could define the terms of the relationship on the basis of what
the fathers purchased for their adult child, as in Meredith's case,
where her father plainly did not know how to relate to her as a young
woman:

When I was younger, my father, brother and I . . . would
go hiking, we'd do a lot of activities together, but as I
started becoming a young woman, my father didn't
know how to relate to me. . . . I can even remember when
I was in my twenties, he would buy me gifts, he would
buy things that were really inappropriate, they were like
childish things. It was like, in his head, I never grew up.

Meredith's father was unable to relate to her basically because of the separation between the sexes that occurs when sexist ideology thrives and is reinforced via ideological socialization; his self was defined in terms of seperateness from, rather than connection with, others, including his daughter. Disjuncture between the sexes is inevitable when boys and girls are raised by their mothers in the absence of their fathers under a patriarchal system, and this disjuncture includes fathers and daughters.

The way fathers have related to the females in the family has prevailed as a source of major irritation in the intergenerational relationship. In one instance, Dan disclosed his dissatisfaction with how his father treated his mother, referring to one recent event:

> If my folks are sitting there at a table eating some dinner, he'll [the father] ask or say, "[Wife], could you please get me a glass of milk." And my mom will put down her fork and get him a glass of milk. When I was down visiting them the last time, for some reason that irked me, that just got under my skin. And it was something that I never mentioned to them.

Earlier in the interview, Dan had made these observations about his mother:

> She's played the housewife raising (his brother) and me. Which is kind of unfortunate, she has a lot of potential. But she was pretty tied up in traditional roles, and I guess that's one reason why I tend to dislike traditional roles. I see it as very stagnant. I wish that my mom would have done more with her life than be a housewife, she's always been very docile, and I'm sorry about that . . . . One real bummer is that my mom was so dependent, and this is what really irks me, she just accepted her housewife role . . . . I always thought she had the potential to make it on her own, but she was just so traditional.

Similarly, Hannah, the daughter of a Jewish couple living in Brooklyn, gave the following deposition in response to the question about having ill feelings toward her parents:

I guess you could call it ill feelings. I have regrets . . . I think that as much as I do love my father, I think that in a lot of ways he's a very stubborn man. And I think that his stubbornness, his insistence on living his business life a certain way, has kind of made life a lot harder on my mother . . . . And it seems he has a greater sense of responsibility toward his business and the people who are working for him than he did for my mother . . . . I do feel a certain amount of anger with him about that.

And the ill feelings I have with my mother is that she's one of those persons who isn't terribly self-confidant. So she hides and doesn't push . . . . I want so much for her to enjoy life and she's so passive . . . . It seems very odd to me because she has such an inward lust that not to act on it—I have a difficult time understanding it.

Sharon, the stepdaughter of a Pentecostal minister, had a much more extreme situation to face than the daughter of the Jewish parents, and spoke of her "extreme hatred" of the way her mother's life has turned out, a circumstance she blames on her stepfather:

I don't believe my mother is living a full life. I think she is psychologically coerced and it's making her physically sick. That bothers me. I feel that it's a loss of a human being's life . . . . Even her mental capacity—not that she is losing it—but she is like stagnating. She's a very intelligent woman as I remember even though she didn't go to college. But now . . . the environment that she lives in is so closed.

As a consequence of her mother's marriage, Sharon has distanced herself emotionally and physically from her mother.

Diane, a Pentecostal herself, has similarly witnessed the psychological coercion of her mother by her stepfather:

When I was growing up, living with my stepfather, my mother was always very weak-willed, and I think she's been unhappy for a real long time and that came out against the kids. She was spiteful, she'd be back-biting,

and she drinks so that compounds the problem. My
mother and I got along a lot better after I moved out.
Now we get along fine.

Now that Diane's stepfather is dead, her mother lives with her.
Looking back, Diane can vividly remember how her mother mis-
treated her, but she says she understands because it was her mother's
own "anger and unhappiness and frustration that made her do this."

The insecurities of traditional mothers manifested themselves in
a variety of ways, one of which was in mothers being jealous of their
daughters. Meredith told how for many years she denied having any
problems in her relationship with her parents, preferring to think that
"We were just one big, happy family." But recently, Meredith has
begun an honest search to identify the sources that squelched the
perfect familial scenario in order to satisfy her need for a truer
representation of her earlier home life. Her mother's jealousy is one
such source:

As I moved into adolescence, my mother and I got into
a lot of conflict of honest competition. My mother
would do things like as family members would come up
to me and tell me how pretty I was, my mother would
say, "Oh, don't tell her that, it will swell her head." She
didn't want anyone to compliment me. I feel like her
own self-image got washed over me, because she projected a lot of her stuff onto me.

Another example of a mother's insecurity adversely affecting
the intergenerational relationship comes from Michael. His reply to
the ill feeling question rested on how he found himself in the
awkward position of being his mother's confidant, in part because
his parents were having difficulty in their marriage:

I had a weird couple of years with my mother, at least I
thought they were strange . . . . She was very depressed
. . . slept a lot, wasn't terribly positive. And I don't think
that she was getting along terribly well with my father,
and I seem to have taken on the role of confidant, and she
would tell me that nobody liked her.

The pain of a mother's exclusion from the life of her husband and how the emotional pattern is passed down to the next generation was beautifully expressed by Elizabeth:

> I also can see and feel intensely the pain that my mother feels . . . my father never having time to do things with her, spend quality time with her . . . . I feel that pain for my mother, because I have a similar situation with a husband who virtually has no time for me . . . . I guess it frightens me and I see this situation as something that could be a repeat with myself being one of the players in twenty-five years. As they say, "The sins of the father are the sins of the sons."

The emotional dependence of mothers on the baby boomers later in life was not all that unique. The reactions of the baby boomers toward their mothers' emotional needs, though, were obviously varied, ranging from feelings of discomfort to compassion.

Sexist ideology is to bear on the circumstance of the baby boomers' mothers in the cases of Dan, Hannah, Sharon, Diane, Meredith, and Michael. Relegated to child rearing and household activities in a society that regards this work as inconsequential to economic exchange and thus trivial, the baby boomers' mothers are suffering from and showing the signs of second-class citizenry. Everything from the mothers' servitude, poor self-image, lack of self-confidence, abuse of their children, and jealousy of their daughters to their emotional dependence on their children reflects the ugliness of capitalist patriarchy.

Passages from the interviews tell of a longing for more loving and caring familial relationships and of an aching consciousness over their lack within the families of orientation. The baby boomers have identified the traditional situation—a tough situation for op-pressed spirits to transcend because of the expectations and the dependencies forced upon them—as the immediate malefactor behind domestic misery. From the iciness, inattention, disillusion-ment, and suppressed potential, to the insecurities, the realities in the everyday life of the baby boomers that stifle happiness among family members have been formed by traditional sex roles. These sex roles are by-products of a particular social arrangement; more specifically, the given situation is a consequence of the larger forces of domination under advanced capitalist patriarchy.

After all, the separation between work and home, the accompanying deep parental love, intense emotional bonding between parents and their children, and income and age and sex stratificationion, are, as critical theorists have established, the handiwork of a system bent on gargantuan profit and the exaltation of the "father-right." Closeness between family members has become associated with dependency. The general structure of love and authority in the privatized family narrows the ties that bind to the ties of economic reliance; thus, closeness can have less to do with interaction and more to do with materialism.

The bonding between the baby boomers and their parents was established without the emotional needs of the children being satisfied. Traditional home life did not create the "one big happy family" scenario. Instead it created dependents, mothers and children, whose emotional needs were often tossed to the wayside in the drive toward dominance and materialism among the fathers. This was cultivated by a larger structure that provided greater financial opportunities (and thus power) to men than women, disparaged the domestic domain where women were assigned, and encouraged the purchasing of goods to keep the bottom line swelling in the black. As a consequence, what usually became more pervasive within the family than "the emotional" was the ability of fathers to provide, or in some cases to have the intent to provide, for the material well-being of the family.

This explains why the baby boomers are still undeniably bonded to the men who so often paid so little attention to them and their mothers, but who did pay the bills and in the best of situations bought them umpteen pairs of shoes and a little sports car. And while the baby boomers wish that their fathers had been more demonstrative in showing their love for them, and wish their fathers would have tried more to understand them as individuals, and wish the relationships they have with their fathers today were more profound than is the case, they also find themselves intricately tied to their fathers. And it explains why the baby boomers who did not receive much financial support from their fathers do not feel close to their fathers. Plus it explains why individuals in our society have come to feel intensely loyal to structures of all shapes and sizes that have not catered to their emotional needs but that have provided them with some degree of material security.

Furthermore, it explains why the emotional needs and social positions of mothers ended up on back burners, resulting in insecurities and other personal deficits. While the traditional arrangement reinforces the larger social order by perpetuating hierarchical relations on a smaller scale, it clearly injures the freedom and personal development of mothers, as well as tranquillity and harmony on the domestic front. The fact that some of the baby boomers were awake to this issue of oppression is encouraging.

Finally, included in this explanation of why the baby boomers feel close or bonded to their parents, yet wish their fathers had been more loving toward them and wish their mothers had been more self-reliant, is something specifically resulting from the mixed feelings: ambivalence. The ambivalence is the infant of ideological socialization, and it is directed not only outward toward the parents but also inward as the baby boomers grapple with their own identities and desires for something more humane than the sex roles they have inherited via ideological socialization.

Chapter 7 THE FORGIVENESS FACTOR

The lack of closeness, the ill feelings, and all the other negative aspects of the intergenerational relationship voiced by the baby boomers were tempered to some degree by the offsprings' tremendous feelings of love, compassion, and consideration toward their older parents. The closing comments of the interviewed typically included a "but" clause. For example:

—"I would say honestly that there are some [ill feelings], but they're tempered with the realization that we are all human. They went through their traumas and have been scared by them, so I don't, I can't say that I bear them."—Shira

—"I suppose I have ill feelings about my parents like everybody does, but I also can qualify them or justify them knowing where they are coming from."—Chris

—"I feel my parents did the best that they could, kind of a copout."—Dan

—"They're parents, what do you expect?"—Anna

One way of qualifying the ill feelings was by attributing parental behavior to a historical epoch. Jane found this answer to the question of whether she had ill feelings toward her parents:

> Yes, in that as I said there were so many things that they
> did that I'm working hard not to do . . . . As I look back
> at those things I understand that they reared us in a
> different time period. Some of those things were very
> well accepted . . . you were a negligent parent if you
> didn't spank them for misbehavior in those days....They
> did what they thought was best at the time, what they felt
> was most appropriate . . . as much as I disagree with that.

Similarly, Nancy explained that while in the past she had some ill feelings toward her parents, more along the line of resentment, she no longer clings to the negative, knowing now that her parents' behavior reflected their life experiences:

> I think after the war he was affected by it and that was his way of dealing with or not dealing with reality to a degree, to stay on the road. And, maybe my mother has the same problem with drinking . . . . I'm sure it has had its affect on me to a large degree. But, it's nothing I can't overcome myself. I mean I can't blame them, they're only human.

The theme in both Jane's and Nancy's cases is that, basically, their parents were products of their time and, for this reason, should be forgiven. After all, they did the best they could under the circumstances. What stands out from these two interviews is the importance of the intergenerational relationship to the baby boomers. The women appreciate their parents' efforts to do their best for them; they feel that their parents love them and care about them, and Jane and Nancy feel the same about their parents.

Along the same lines, some baby boomers talked about how they wished things were different between them and their parents, but they are not. Their parents try to do their best, though their best is not always constructive, as attested by Maria:

> They've done the best that they can for me. Generally, we don't get along. In passing, I wish we did, I wish we were like a television family, but we're not. Partly my personality, too. But I know they did the best that they could. They want the best for me and they tried.
>
> Certainly there are things that they've done and are doing and will do in the future that will make me angry . . . [but] I think they have always done the best they've been able to do. My mother sometimes says that she doesn't think she was a very good parent to me, and I think that what she wants is reassurance from me that that's not true. And I've never had any trouble giving

her that reassurance because I really do feel that she's
done the absolute best she can.

Wishing to be like a "television family" is certainly a product of
its time. Baby boomers like Maria were the first generation of
children to grow up watching programs on television. They watched
perfect family after perfect family flutter across the screen, measures of domesticity sure to leave many of the young fans disappointed with their own home situations which, unlike Hollywood's
families, were real. Can you imagine the children watching "Leave
It to Beaver" or "The Donna Reed Show" and then comparing their
own lives to such perfection? On television, the and cars were always new; parents were always calm, content, pleasing, and willing
to interact with their children and happily in love with one another;
and children were always respectful to their parents and never did
anything outside the norm of mainstream American society. Everyone looked great—the highly touted "All American Family," which
in reality rarely if ever existed.

So it is not surprising to find Maria saying she wishes her family
were more like a television family, though it is not. It is also not
startling to learn that Maria's mother needs reassurance from time
to time that she was, in fact, a good mother. Remember, she watched
the television programs too. Plus, Maria's mother's role demand
specified that she be a "perfect mother." Here, the issue is the
standardization of perfection under a particular social arrangement,
and the consequence is feeling inadequate and the need for both
child and parent to accept one another as well as their own family in
spite of socially defined imperfections. Part of maturity, according
to many of the baby boomers, is accepting parents for who they are.
A quote from Rita sums up this sentiment:

No, I learned a long time ago to acknowledge them for
the human beings that they are. I gave up my childhood
pettiness of needing them to be someone I need them to
be. Basically, I grew up.

Rita is a professor of psychology living in the Northeast who
grew up in Oklahoma on her parents' ranch. Her mother was a
lifelong schoolteacher; her father, a rancher who finished "maybe

the fifth grade," was educated the "Cherokee way." Her father "is a more traditional, conservative, patriarchical variety," and Rita's mother is "strongly religious." These characteristics combined with Rita's "genius and wild-child curious" created some family feuds during Rita's teen and early adulthood years. Today, Rita spends every summer with her parents, helping them with the ranch. There was a time in her adult years, though, when Rita did not make it back home to see her parents.

> The honest answer is that I got myself exiled for about five years for differences of opinion [from her father]. And I saw that my life was going by and there was no way to replace those years. So I went home and made peace.

This event happened when Rita was in her early twenties. Today, Rita feels close to her parents, closer to her mother, for she has always been her mother's "favorite kid." Rita and her father have "an Indian standoff" meaning there are certain things they just do not discuss, since neither one is going to change. The standoff is for the sake of closeness, the recognized part of the relationship that truly matters to them.

Acceptance of parents was equally important to Suzanne and Joyce, who took the approach of taking the good with the bad. Said Suzanne:

> With my mother, she's just my mother. You take the good with the bad, realizing she's just a human being like everybody else. That she's not beyond being incapable of making mistakes.

And Joyce noted:

> My father, on the other hand, has always been kind of abrasive in his relationship with me. Therefore I don't really have that good of feeling toward him, although I'm not trying to carry a chip on my shoulder about him anymore. I just try and take him as he is and accept what he is and try to see the good things about him rather than

the bad things. Anymore, we don't have that much time together to carry ill feelings around about our parents.

"Life is too short, life goes on, and besides, I've grown up and accepted my parents," is the line that sums up not only Suzanne's and Joyce's feelings but Stella's as well.

Stride and maturity, these were the concepts behind Stella's change of heart toward her mother. Stella is a black woman who was raised until age twelve by her aunt and uncle and then given over to her mother, who was an incorrigible, angry young person lacking education, income, and social skills. Stella's mother abused her both physically and mentally for many years. In spite of the beatings, name-calling, the time her mother tried to have her kicked out of nursing school even though she was maintaining a B average, the times her mother chased her friends away from the house, or the time her mother falsely accused her of sleeping with her stepfather, Stella says she feels close to her mother and does not harbor bitter feelings toward her:

> I think what it is, I have matured. I can understand her now. Number one, I can understand her resentment and anger. She didn't get the education, but she blamed it on me. This is what I tell her, "I didn't tell you to lay down with my father, did I? That was your mistake."
>
> I wouldn't say I had any ill feelings. I think I feel more sympathy . . . . Bitterness, no. I think because . . . she learned to accept me as an adult, and she knows I mean what I say. Like I'll tell her now, "Go to hell." I mean it now, and see, she has no control over me now and she used to have.

Again, here is a situation of both child and parent understanding family history and wanting acceptance in spite of it all. The past, a combination of racism, capitalism, and patriarchy, is not pretty, but it has been privately shared by the two. They have each other; at times that may not have been much, but at least it was something. For those who have little in a world wrought with plenty, having each other can mean a lot.

While parents may have their share of bad qualities, they also have good qualities that are worth remembering, according to many baby boomers, including Les:

> Basically, you just have to accept people as to what they are and . . . accept my father as who he was and my mom. Now, if they were complete strangers, I might have less to do with them . . . but since they raised you, you also know the very good qualities that they have as parents.

And like so many baby boomers, Les looks back to the past with compassionate eyes, seeing what was and why it was that way:

> Well, my dad was pretty critical growing . . . when I was a child. Yet, a lot of that was his way and I think if he had, if he could do it over, he would. He made mistakes as a parent, and I don't fault him for that. Actually, I should say "no" to the question. I don't have any ill feelings. That I understand those much more now than I did when I was younger.

Other baby boomers just looked at the past as "history" to be forgotten: "It happened, it is over, nothing can change it, so let it rest." Such is the situation with Ellen. She used to be troubled by the fact that her father was a mechanical engineer who worked on nuclear weapons, but now she focuses on his good qualities such as his intellect, and she sets aside that what she dislikes about him:

> My father was a mechanical engineer for . . . a federal government agency . . . where they engineer most of the nuclear weapons for this country . . . . I think I had kind of a traditional father/daughter thing going where . . . my dad was just great, basically I liked him a lot, except this thing about his occupation and that really bothered me . . . . Back to this stuff about working things out with my father, I still don't approve . . . . But I still love my father, I respect his intellect, I respect the way he makes decisions, and I wish he hadn't done that for his job, but, I mean, he did.

Focusing more on the intergenerational relationship than on her parent's occupation as Ellen, Elizabeth spoke at length about how she has come to accept her mother and to push the unpleasant out of her mind:

> With my mother, the relationship is a little bit patho-logical, and it's been hurtful, but that's water under the bridge, and that's something I would have preferred that we could have healed and possibly grown together in our relationship, but . . . . Of course, everything good about me is because of my parents. And that's something that is equally important. No parent is perfect. I am certainly not a perfect parent . . . . I guess when I look back on my parents' relationship and our home life, I can see where the big problems were and big flaws were.

> Because Elizabeth is able to keep in perspective the pains of the past, she is able to maintain a close rela-tionship with her parents that carries over into the grandchild/grandparent relationship: I always look forward to seeing my parents when they come to visit or when I go to visit them, because I see how my mother enjoys it. She enjoys talking with me, and she especially enjoys talking with the children.

Still, Elizabeth keeps a distance between herself and her parents, for she believes that if she were to see her parents on a day-to-day basis, the past would come back to haunt her and infringe on the warmth that has been established in the familial relationship:

> So I would have to say that I love my parents very much, and I feel very close to them, although I could never survive seeing them daily and being totally immersed in their day-to-day problems. It would be too much for me because it would be a reminder of the problems, the shortcomings in our home as we were growing up.

In contrast, the past was something some of the baby boomers wanted to know more about, particularly in terms of family heritage.

The interest in family history created a link between the baby boomers and their parents, one that made it easier for them to talk to their parents and feel connected to them. Connie, a professor with an Asian background, had such a link:

> But I think in the last few years I've felt interested in my mother and more interested in her parents, in family as a large-scale thing. And it has led me to be very curious anyway, but since it is a closed door now all of a sudden I want to get through it. Where we were never interested in any of that stuff when we were growing up, we'd go, "Oh Chinese, *uck!*" So, I think I'm more curious about their backgrounds. I think that's natural too, as your parents get older you want to save some part of what they are, have some of those memories.

Saving a part of who your parents are by learning of their past brushes on the subjects of interconnectedness from one generation to another and on immortality. Connie clearly values her family affiliation and desires to be part of it. She also shows a strong desire to keep the familial heritage alive, the essence of her parents and herself. From Connie's perspective, this is "natural" and perhaps to a certain extent it is, but it is also accentuated by the social organization under which Connie lives, which, as critical theorists have shown, privatizes the family, making for acute dependency and bonding.

Family connections were carried forward as well; the baby boomers were likely to take past family mistakes into consideration in rearing their own children. Consequently, many baby boomers with children, while forgiving of their parents, added a clause pertaining to how they are making a conscious effort to be different from their parents in rearing their own children. The following excerpt from Elizabeth's interview is a good example:

> I have a much stronger desire to make things different for my children and for myself. I'm certainly not satisfied with the situation in my own household with my children and my husband. I also realize that there are limitations when you're dealing with another, the other spouse being totally unreceptive and unwilling to listen

and try and change the things that I find very hurtful and inappropriate. I often think to myself that my goal as a parent is to help my children grow up to be fulfilled and attain a lot more of their potential than I did and to help them not have to go through the emotional problems I have in my own life.

Elizabeth has brought up some telling points here. For one, she is deliberately trying to rear her two daughters differently from the way her parents reared her. But, her efforts are blunted by her husband's insensitivity regarding this issue. The old way dies hard, especially for those who have the most to gain from the status quo. Given the familial structure under advanced capitalism, which places wives and children in subordinate positions due to economics, it is not surprising that Elizabeth wishes for change, not her husband. And under the current structure, Elizabeth is the parent who was socialized, thanks to her sex, to be conscious and caring about the emotional well-being of her children, whereas her husband was socialized to think in terms of individual success. As Chodorow (1978) claimed, the different socialization of the sexes produces tension between the sexes. In this case, the tension is intensified by the fact that both children are both female.

One question remains: Why is Elizabeth seeking change instead of maintaining the traditional family structure? Turning to what Marx said about emancipation is a good starting point for answering this question. According to Marx and Engels (1848), there is a point at which contradiction becomes so prevalent that the oppressed become conscious of their situation, unite, and overthrow the old order. Over the past few decades, women in the United States have begun to wake up to their second-class standing in society, as contradictions between traditional expectations and contemporary realities intensify. One by one, women have joined together to fight patriarchy. It is not a revolution in Marx's sense, but it is a movement that seeks to change the social order.

The home is not the haven it is purported to be, nor is it a realm in which women are totally satisfied, as Lasch (1977) and many feminists have said. But it is, as Elshtain (1981) maintains, one of only a few spots in a capitalist patriarchal society where the individual can feel a sense of belonging and emotional ties. The contradictions began in the nineteenth century when women found themselves devoted to child rearing even though they were better educated than ever before in history. Women were both exalted and degraded, fulfilled and incensed, useful and ornamental, isolated and visible in a social world that took for granted the radical separation between the private and the public. The contradictions mounted in the youth of the baby boomers as women entered universities and the job market in droves, as women's incomes became necessary for family survival, as women's rights became linked to the high ideals of human and civil rights that became more pronounced through the unveiling of public lies surrounding Vietnam, race riots, and Watergate. Ultimately, the contradictions undermined blind faith in the absolute authority of the powers-that-be in American society.

Part of the emotional pattern seen in the present-day American family reflects a strong desire on the part of adult children to maintain intergenerational harmony by forgiving all that their parents have (willingly or not) spoiled—perhaps it is an unconscious way of lessening the ambivlence or a way of making it more palatable. Whatever, the forgiveness is understandable in a social environment where the family unit is extremely privatized, existing (1) without everyday support from a community of other women and men and (2) within a larger structure where competition reigns over cooperation. Simply, the environment has been conducive to a deep child/parental bonding and to care and coziness having been relegated to the private realm. Adult children love their parents and need their parents to love them, no question about it. But there is also no question about the social demands magnifying the basic bond between child and parent.

What the forgiveness factor represents in the larger design of social relations is how, as a people, Americans have adapted to oppression by first accepting human arrangements as they exist and then seeking justifications for injustices and inadequacies. The thought that some greater source is behind the ills of human relationships ceases to enter most people's minds as they are preoccupied with the here and now, striving to find some expression of joy and security in a not so joyful and secure society. And, the striving is enhanced by societal notions that emotional fulfillment should be satisfied within the home among loved ones and belongings. It is all a part of the American dream.

Possibilities

But the American dream has dissipated somewhat as contradictions force its fabrications to the forefront of our critical consciousness. Baby boomers are questioning the old structure and trying to find new ways to enhance relations inside and outside the home. The task of social scientists is to answer questions and present solutions about how to create better social relations in American society. Information gathered from interviews with baby boomers aids in our understanding of the strain in the adult child/parent relationship and how to improve relations in our families and our larger social structure. The goal necessitates the eradication of oppressive relations.

As a starting point, obtaining the goal would require a new attitude about respectability, especially in terms of sexual differentiation. Inhibitions about nudity and about bodily functions, sounds, and pleasures would need to be diminished. Instead of denying our humanness, we would want to celebrate it. We, as parents, would regard the rearing of children as an important feature of parenthood for both women and men; and in our child rearing, we would need to stop forcing our children to choose between personal gratification and our affection. Certainly it would be important to rethink the notion of punishment altogether, realizing that guidance need not be induced by threats or acts of violence.

Neither father-right nor mother-right would prevail in our homes; each implies abuses of power within the family. Our attitude would be one of individual-right guaranteed to parents and children alike. We would understand the difference between guidance and control, practicing the former to the best of our abilities.

We would also need to stop and reevaluate communication between ourselves and our children, keeping in mind that "knowledge is power." Freer-spirited parents would not feel threatened by open and shared communication with their children, nor would they make a distinction between the parents' world and the children's world; the understanding would be that parents and children live in one world. Efforts would be made to inform and explain, rather than hoard the understandings of life, and in this way substantive conversations could begin early in the intergenerational relationship. In the new situation, there would not be any secrets, for what would there be to hide? We hide what we are ashamed of, and shame is grounded in social expectations and ideas about appropriateness, both of which would be redefined.

As liberated parents, we would cheer our female and male children's voicings, urging them to express themselves verbally, artistically, physically and through any other medium of their choice; we would likewise teach our children about social tolerance and about horizontal thinking. And we would want our feelings toward our children and their feelings toward us to be heard through the spoken and written word, through embraces and smiles, through tender considerations in everyday life. In our efforts to eradicate domination from our home lives, we would stop expecting our children to be clones of ourselves and begin viewing their uniqueness as something to rejoice about.

Human happiness in this situation would not be derived from another pair of jeans or another video cassette, but through having reached one's full potential. As individuals, we would want to nurture creativity, inquisitiveness, and physical fitness in our children and in ourselves—and restrictions by age and sex would be taboo. Success would be gauged by human happiness instead of gross income, color of occupational collar, or utilitarian productivity. In this way, we would encourage our children to think about who and what they want to be and then accept the choices they make for themselves. Our participation in our children's lives would be in the name of companionship, period. We would not want to be a force for our children to reckon with, but a force in which they would find strength and courage.

And coupled with the changes at home would be moves toward converting the larger social structure into a more humane structure, meaning a less authoritarian and hierarchical one. Obviously, laws would have to change, as would the role of the state; our political system would need revamping along with our economic system. Our societal values of rivalry, consumption, and competition would need to be replaced with peace, frugality, and community (a suggestion proposed by Luc Versteylen, a Jesuit teacher in Belgium, on how to better our social and spiritual selves). Historically, these latter values have not been compatible with monopoly capitalism.

The dream is that a freer society would be created through a process in which there would be an interplay between modifications in both the individual and the social organization of the society,

culminating in a political philosophy preserving the well-being of all
life on this planet. With ideological socialization abolished and the
institutionalization of nonauthoritarian, nonhierarchical relations,
individuals, freed from ambivalence, would define their own des-
tinies, achieve their potentialities, consider new possibilities, improve
their spiritual selves, and always question their social relations. One
consequence of the freer existence would be better relations between
adult children and their parents; another would be that notions of
filial adaptation would become history.

PART II

BABY BOOMERS' AMBIVLENCE: QUANTITATIVE FINDINGS

Chapter 8   MAINSTREAM RESEARCH ON INTERGENERATIONAL RELATIONS

In contrast to critical works, dominant research on the adult child/parent relationship ignores the social organization of society. It covers a wide range of topics, each having in common the issue of filial adaptation. Explanations of filial adaptation take into account the factors that both bind and break intergenerational ties in the United States, but generally do so without reference to capitalist patriarchy. The first part of this chapter is devoted to reviewing what has been said about the binding factors of the intergenerational relationship, the second to the trends believed to be affecting it, and the third and final part to the noted strains in the contemporary American adult child/parent relationship.

Binding Factors of the Intergenerational Relationship

Affectional Bond: The "Close" Factor

The affectional bond between adult children and parents is usually cited as the primary factor governing close intergenerational relationships (Cicirelli 1983; Johnson and Bursk 1977; Streib 1965). Although difficult to define, the affectional bond is usually identified with positive sentiments of love, respect, appreciation, and the feeling of attachment people have for one another (Bengston and Schrader 1981; Bowlby 1979; Quinn 1984). It is expressed by association and protective behaviors.

Concern over the affirmation of the affectional bond is apparent by the numerous studies that have been conducted on this topic. For example, in a national survey on the degree of interaction between generations, Shanas (1977) found that 52 percent of her respondents reported seeing at least one of their children in the previous twenty-four hours. Harris and Associates (1975) found as high as 85 percent of the older sample had seen one or more of their children within the the past week or two. As many as 56 percent of Mexican-Americans, 40 percent of Anglos, and 33 percent of Blacks reporting interaction with their adult children sometime during the previous day in Bengston and Manuel's (1976) study of a Los Angeles community. In another cross-ethnic survey, Cantor (1975) found that half of her sample of older New Yorkers saw their children at least once a week.

Cicirelli (1983) thinks the affectional bond is not necessarily enunciated by acts of daily contact or personal intimacy, but is definitely proclaimed by periodic (on the average once a week) visits and telephone calls, in addition to letter writing and protective behaviors such as providing physical or financial assistance to the member in need. Bowlby (1979) argues that the affectional bond remains strong throughout the family life cycle. The family bond is favored over friendship by Troll and Smith (1976), who see it as being based more on obligation than on shared interests.

The point stressed by social gerontologists is that the affectional bond is still expressed in the adult child/parent relationship. Treas and Bengston (1987), however, identify four factors of social differentiation affecting the nature of contact between generations: sex, martial status, social class, and ethnicity. It seems that daughters more than sons, unmarried children more than married ones, working-class offspring more than children of other social classes, the upwardly mobile son rather than the downwardly mobile one, and Mexican American children more than either blacks or whites have closer contact with their parents (Adams 1968; Hill et al. 1970; Lopata 1979; Sussman 1965).

Filial Responsibility: The "Caring" Factor

Filial responsibility is the factor most often identified with adult children having a caring relationship with parents. By filial responsibility, researchers generally mean the obligations adult children have in meeting their aging parents' needs. It includes maintaining contact with parents and seeing to their well-being, if needed, by helping them with household tasks, finances, errands, health care, social contacts, and psychological soundness (Scelbach 1984;

Sussman 1965; Treas and Bengston 1987). Noting that adult children are becoming more involved in assisting their parents with bureaucratic paperwork than with other responsibilities, Seelbach (1984) created the term contemporary filial responsibility.

Filial responsibility in the United States has been traced to the Judeo-Christian admonition to "Honor thy father and thy mother (Linzer 1986; Seelbach 1984), the early socialization of the child (Silverstone and Hyman 1976; Woehrer 1982), and the ethnic family structure (Woehrer 1982). Boszormenyi-Nagy and Spark (1973) have proposed that because adult children feel indebted to their parents, they are compelled to satisfy family traditions of filial responsibility. Beyond a sense of indebtedness, filial responsibility has been associated with mutual aid (Johnson and Bursk 1977).

Social support is another aspect of filial responsibility. As defined by Gottlieb, social support consists of "verbal and/or nonverbal information or advice, tangible aid, or action that is proffered by social intimatesor inferred by their presence and has beneficial emotional or behavioral effects on the recipient" (1983, 28). Social support is a significant resource linked to improving health outcomes (Gottlieb 1981), buffering depression and anxiety (LaRocco et al. 1980), increasing life satisfaction and happiness (Gottlieb 1981), and enhancing self-esteem (Pearline et al. 1981). In his study of the elderly, Gottlieb concludes that the morale of older people is increased by social support from family, friends, and neighbors.

The exchange of assistance and support between adult children and their parents is well documented in the literature (Cantor 1975; Lopata 1973; Rosow 1967; Seelbach 1977; Sussman 1965; Treas 1977; Troll et al. 1979). For example, as early as 1965, Sussman saw that older parents preferred to rely on their families rather than public agencies for assistance. A study by Rosow in 1967 revealed that working-class parents are more likely to be recipients of material support than middle-class parents, who are more inclined to receive moral support from their adult children. In 1975, Cantor found the family to be the primary source of social support for older parents living in New York. Another study showed that the more vulnerable the parents, the more likely they are to receive aid from their children (Seelbach 1977). Shanas (1980) reported that seven out of ten parents aged sixty-five and over survey give and receive help from their children.

The subject of filial responsibility is bound to the norms of women and domestics. Lopata (1970) disclosed that daughters are more likely than sons to provide emotional and daily support to an older parent, and that daughters are the ones who typically end up taking widowed mothers and mothers-in-law into their homes. Lopata (1973) also revealed that the daughters of widows in the Chicago area were more likely to take direct care of their mothers, whereas sons handled financial affairs and funeral arrangements. Cantor (1980) too found daughters to be the primary caretakers of older parents. Treas and Bengston summed up the situation by referring to women as the "mainstay of family support for the aged" (1987,633). Social gerontologists recognize that aspects of modern life in the United States can obstruct the willingness and the capability of some adult children to maintain the affectional bond and meet their filial obligations. Notable trends in filial adaptation can be seen by looking at the records of the U.S. *Statistical Abstracts* and the U.S. Senate Special Committee on Aging, and examining the way in which the data have been interpreted by mainstream social gerontologists.

Statistics

Population Trends

America is aging. The life expectancy of Americans at birth has increased about thirty years over the past century (*Statistical Abstract* 1987, 69). In 1900, only 1 in 25 Americans was age 65 years and over; today the ratio is closer to 1 in 8; while the population 65 years and older constituted only 4 percent of the total population in 1900, today that figure has jumped to about 12 percent (*Developments in Aging* 1985,1; *Statistical Abstract* 1987,18). At the turn of the twentieth century, there were more than 4.9 million older Americans; in 1985 there were more than 28.5 million (Developments in Aging, 1985: 11; *Statistical Abstract* 1987,18). Even more astounding is the fact that our senior population has grown twice as fast as the rest of the population over the past two decades. Among the Americans 65 years of age and over, more and more are living well into their 80s and 90s, in fact, the 85-plus population is the fastest-growing age group, thanks to improved health care (*Developments in Aging* 1985,13).

Aging as a Women's Issue. Many older Americans are women: Life expectancy for women has improved threefold over that for men in the past forty years. In 1985, there were 5.5 million more elderly women than men, a considerable change from 1960 when the difference was 1.6 million. After age 85, this disparity is more marked, from 67 men per 100 women in 1960 to only 40 men per 100 women in 1984 (*Developments in Aging* 1985,16).

Generations Growing Old Together. The age distance between adjacent generations is declining; the distance has dropped from 30 years in 1900 to approximately 20 years at present. What with life expectancy increasing and distance between generations dropping, it is becoming commonplace for "children" in their 60s and 70s to have living parents (*Developments in Aging* 1985,14).

Fewer Siblings. While elders, many of whom are women, are increasing per family, children are fewer and are born closer together today than in decades past. Each successive generation of women since 1900 has given birth to fewer children. In 1957, the total fertility rate was 3.8 children per woman; by 1973, the total fertility rate stood at a low level of 1.9 children per woman; and the rate has fluctuated little ever since (*Statistical Abstract* 1987,58).

Social Trends

Women in the Paid Work Force. Over the past few decades, women have been entering the paid work force in ever increasing numbers. Fifty years ago, about 27 percent of American women were in the paid labor force; now, the figure is closer to 55 percent (*Statistical Abstract* 1987,382–383). Furthermore, some 68 percent of women working outside the home have children ages 6 to 13; nearly 54 percent have children under 6 years of age, and approximately 50 percent of all married women with infants are in the civilian labor force (*Statistical Abstract* 1987,383).

Marital Arrangements and Disruptions. Staying single, divorce, dual-career marriage, and single parenthood have increased among Americans in recent decades. In 1970, 13.7 percent of females and 18.9 percent of males never married, compared to 18.2 percent and

25.2 percent, respectively, in 1985 (*Statistical Abstract* 1987,39). The percentage of the adult population divorced rose from 3.9 to 8.7 for females and 2.5 to 6.5 for males between 1970 and 1985 (*Statistical Abstract* 1987,38). Dual-earner families have become the norm as married women have entered the paid labor force: in 1986, 55 percent of the female labor force was married, in contrast to only 16.7 percent in 1940 (*Statistical Abstract* 1987,382). The proportion of American families headed by a single female parent was 19.3 percent in 1985, nearly double that of 1970 (*Statistical Abstract* 1987,49).

Geographic Mobility. Geographic mobility, or internal migration, is high in the United States. Within the five year period from 1980 to 1985, 39.9 percent of civilian Americans moved at least once (*Statistical Abstract* 1987,25). The older population is least likely to move. Of the persons who moved between 1982 and 1983, only 4.9 percent were older persons (*Developments in Aging* 1985,28). But, the number of older persons changing residence is increasing; there was a 50 percent jump in state-to-state migration among older Americans in the 1970s compared to the 1960s (*Developments in Aging* 1985, 28–29).

Economic Trends

Over the past century, America has changed from a basically rural, agricultural, competitive capitalist society to a predominately urban, postindustrial, monopoly capitalist society. It has been transformed from a society using simple technologies to one using sophisticated technologies mainly for productive profit and military supremacy.

The Great Depression to the Present. The monopolistic practices of overexpansion financed through credit borrowing weakened the U.S. economy during the 1920s, until overproduction and falling prices caused the U.S. economy to collapse in 1929 (Palmer and Colton 1971; Piven and Cloward 1982). Three years later, 12 to 14 million Americans were out of work: national income fell to less than half what it had been during 1929; and in another three years, over 50 percent of the population 65 years and over was unemployed (Palmer and Colton 1971). One response by the U.S. government to this problem was the passage of the 1935 Social Security Act (Piven and Cloward 1982).

Social Security changed the economic role of the aged. Since the 1935 act was passed, the participation rate of men 65 and over in the civilian labor force has steadily declined, from nearly 50 percent in 1950 to 15.6 percent in 1985 (*Developments in Aging* 1985,56). The historical trend is more difficult to assess for women given their relatively recent entrance into "employment status." Older women are also underrepresented in the paid labor force; in 1950, the percentage rate was 10, and in 1985 it was 7.1 (*Developments in Aging* 1985,57).

Since 1935, the U.S. government has played an ever-increasing role in supporting its elderly citizens. The percentage of the federal budget spent on the elderly grew from 15 percent in 1960 to 26 percent in 1986; in dollar terms, the increase was from around $43 billion to $269.5 billion (*Developments in Aging* 1985,95). In 1965, Congress passed the Older Americans Act, which included Medicare and other federal programs for the elderly such as housing, energy assistance, and food stamps. The Age Discrimination in Employment Act was passed in 1967 to prohibit the use of age as a criterion for hiring, it was amended in 1978 to raise the age of mandatory retirement from 65 to 70. By 1972, Congress had passed a law for automatic annual cost-of-living increases for Social Security beneficiaries.

Older Americans rely heavily on government support: About 90 percent of retired Americans draw Social Security. In 1984, 38 percent of older Americans' income came from Social Security, and 49 percent of their personal health care expenditures were covered by Medicare. The economic status of the elderly varies dramatically, more so than for any other age group. Some elderly have substantial resources, while others have almost none, the lowest money incomes being among the oldest of the elderly. In 1984, 12.4 percent of older Americans were living at or below poverty level, and the median family income for the elderly population was $18,118—an amount $10,854 less than the median income for families with a head aged 25–64 (*Developments in Aging* 1985,36).

Although the United States pulled through the Great Depression, even experiencing relative prosperity from 1945 to 1970, it has not overcome economic crisis. For example, the outstanding gross national debt rose from $382.6 trillion in 1970 to $1,827.5 trillion in 1985 (*Statistical Abstract* 1987,292). The response of Ronald Reagan's administration in the 1980s: increase retirement age, postpone cost-of-living increases, and raise the senior citizen's share of hospital charges under Medicare.

Economic and state changes have had a direct impact on family structure. Whereas the family was once a producing unit it has now become a consuming unit. Interestingly, one of the arguments presented in favor of Social Security was that it would provide the aged with income with which to buy goods, thereby helping the general economy of the country. While, in the main, both young and old citizens are regarded as "consumers," they are not both regarded as "producers," for this is a status given only to persons in the paid labor force.

The above-mentioned facts and figures certainly do not exhaust all the societal changes that have occurred over the past century in the United States, but they do represent some of the chief changes named by social gerontologists as affecting the adult child/parent relationship.

The Interpretation

Social gerontologists have turned to historically recent trends to explain why the contemporary adult child/parent relationship in the United States is often strained and how the problem can be minimized. Recent trends, taken together, have suggested to some social gerontologists that a dramatic transition in intergenerational relations is stretching the limits of close and caring intergenerational ties.

For example, the cover page of Halpern's *Helping Your Aging Parents* (1987) reads:

> The number of elderly Americans is growing rapidly. People are living longer but tend to develop more chronic illnesses. At the same time, most adult children are now in the workforce and raising children of their own; they have fewer siblings to turn to and less government support. So, although most adult children

care deeply about their aging parents, seeing them
through their later years can be a burden.

As social gerontologists see it, there are more parents, grandparents, and even great-grandparents than ever before in American
history, and more elderly ultimately equals more filial responsibility.
Some scholars (e.g., Townsend 1968), have explained the elder
equation in terms of the family form, suggesting that while in
preindustrial societies the extended family may have had only one
surviving grandparent under its care, nowadays the nuclear family
may have responsibility for as many as four living grandparents plus
one or two great-grandparents. Social gerontoloists often discuss the
special characteristics of the older population. For example, Johnson and Bursk (1977) found the better the parents' health, finances,
and living environments, the better their relationships with their
children. Brody (1981), Korbin (1976), Treas and Bengston (1987),
Steinmetz and Amsden (1983), and Troll (1971) have each called
attention to the growing number of very old family members with
many basic needs. Steinmetz and Amsden strike home this point
when they write that "for the first time in history, there is a large
number of generationally inversed families in which dependent
elders must rely on their kin for prolonged physical, emotional, and
financial aid" (1983,174).

The elders with the greatest needs are typically women. Since
women, in general, live longer, they experience more pain than men
of widowhood and often the sorrow of losing sons. The plight of
widows is worsened by social realities in the United States, including female employment and compensation. Widows typically have
the most needs but the fewest resources (Treas and Bengston 1987).
Widow dependency is an especially acute problem for daughters. It
is they and not sons who usually end up trying to fill-in the deficient
income and other resource gaps of their widowed mothers (Treas
and Bengston 1987). Korbin (1976) is concerned that daughters,
caught between role expectations and the needs of widowed parents,
including in-laws, are finding themselves with responsibilities beyond their personal capabilities. Similarly, Cantor (1980) minds that
the caregivers in her study, mostly women, complained of considerable strain associated with filial responsibilities.

The changing roles of women have been directly related to the elderly dependency equation. Troll (1976) contends that the increase of women in the paid workforce is significant because women are the traditional caretakers of elderly family members. And in a popular work, Brody (1981) warns that many women today are caught in the middle of providing care for both their families of orientation and procreation. Treas (1977) reminds us, too, that whereas in days gone by women, not as bound to the "feminine mystique," were less inclined to marry and have children than their contemporary counterparts; hence, maiden aunts might be around to care for the elders. Brody and Schoonover (1986) discovered that daughters who work outside the home provide less personal care to their older parents than the "nonworking" daughters. Today middle-aged women are worn down by the diverse needs of their loved ones, including aging parents and in-laws.

The stress of multiple roles has been seen by social gerontologists as a problem for both male and female adult children who have the responsibility of caring for their own children, maintaining their jobs, dealing with their own impending retirement and bearing the burden of their parents' problems (Silverstone and Hyman 1976; Steinmetz and Amsden 1983; Sussman 1976; Treas and Bengston 1987). In addition, Cicirelli (1983, 1986) points out that today's middle-aged offspring with marital disruption often have even less time, money, and energy than the rest of the population to maintain close ties with or provide help to their older parents.

The problem of elderly dependency is further compounded by the reality that there are fewer siblings today than in yesteryear to share filial responsibility (Seelbach 1984). Singlehood, single parenting, dual careers, and other alternative lifestyles are accounted for as factors stretching the durability of intergenerational relations (Skolnick and Skolnick 1980; Seelbach 1984).

Being an attached and responsible adult child is also believed to be affected by geographic mobility. Troll (1971) found residential propinquity to play a principal role in the adult child/parent relationship. Cowgill (1974) cited geographic mobility as one of the factors of modernization undermining intergenerational ties. Residential proximity, according to Cicirelli (1983), is greater among adult children who are more attached to their parents. Shanas (1979) wrote, in a discussion of the alienation myth:

Because of the geographic mobility of the population of
the U.S., most old people who have children live at great
distances from their children; Because of the alienation
of old people from their children, most older parents
rarely see their children; Because of the predominance
of the nuclear family in the U.S. most old people rarely
see their siblings or other relatives. . . . Despite what
everyone knows, each of the above hypotheses has been
disproved. In the United States most old people with
children live close to at least one of their children and
see at least one child often. Most old people see their
siblings and relatives often. (1979,6)

Shanas (1973) has maintained, however, that socio-emotional
distance is far more important than geographic distance in gauging
closeness between the generations.

Included in the trends identified by social gerontologists for
interfering with adult children's interpersonal relationships with
their parents are various cultural changes in the United States.
Wynne (1986) cautions that while traditionally the young were
socialized to have a sense of obligation to the aged, today this is no
longer the case. Historical eras are also taken into account by
Deutscher (1987), who attributes some resentment between generations to the sharp contrast in values about money and consumption
patterns of parents who experienced the Great Depression and their
children who did not.

Focusing on adult children exclusively, Skolnick and Skolnick
(1980) suggest that contemporary adult children are faced with the
contradiction of a "morality stressing enjoyment and self-fulfillment
and a morality of duty, responsibility, work, and self-denial." As
Turner (1976) tells us, the 1970s was the "me decade," emphasizing
self-expression. After reading through popular periodicals, Benton
(1981) came to the conclusion that Americans are becoming less
inhibited and concerned with what others expect from them. These
changes led Treas and Bengston (1987) to foretell of the frustration
adult children may experience in caregiving given the newer norms
fostering self-fulfillment. For middle-aged children who have a
commitment to being depended upon by their parents, Blenkner
(1965) has come up with the term *filial maturity*. Historical trends

in the United States have hindered adult children's abilities to meet their filial obligations, a circumstance leading to ill feelings toward parents. Steinmetz and Amsden (1983) write that "feelings of love and respect easily can turn into guilt, hatred, and disappointment as children attempt to function in their next roles of caregiver" (1983,174). Even the anticipation of filial responsibility can be distressing for the middle generation (in particular, for adult children who have not reached a true filial maturity), a phenomenon Cicirelli (1983) calls *filial anxiety*. If there are unresolved interpersonal conflicts between children and older parents, the hurt and bitterness can intensify an already troublesome situation (Simos 1975). Adding another component to filial anxiety, Troll (1986) suggests that adult children, in seeing their parents age and die, may become anxious about their own mortality. At worst, the stress of filial responsibility can lead to elder abuse (Anetzberger 1987; Steinmetz and Amsden 1983).

The degree of ill feelings between adult children and their parents varies by study: Simos (1975) reported only one-fourth of her sample of adult children claimed cordial or warm relationships with their parents; in contrast, Cicirelli (1981) announced as many as 36 percent and 39 percent of his sample of adult children reported no conflict with their mothers and fathers, respectively. Whichever the more accurate estimate, the truth is that there are strains in the adult child/parent relationship.

In summary, it is clear that adult children's feelings toward their parents can range from love and compassion (Seelbach 1984) to ill feelings including a sense of burden, hostility and contempt (Silverstone and Hyman 1976), anxiety (Cicirelli 1983), frustration (Ragan 1979), guilt (Otten and Shelley 1976), strain (Treas and Bengston 1987), and jealousy and insecurity (Seelbach 1984). Since these ill feelings are traced to timely trends, they are assumed to be an unavoidable human condition in modern society.

Certainly, in situations where aging parents are failing in health and resources, needing daily care from one or more of their children, it is understandable that there is strain in the intergenerational relationship. But to generalize this strain to the intergenerational relationship itself is possibly to omit crucial factors surrounding the adult child/parent relationship, and in turn to propose solutions that fail to address root causes behind the problem of intergenerational conflict.

The solutions suggested by the mainstream perspective attempt to minimize the stresses of adult children and help them cope with the problem of parental dependency. At one level, advice is given to adult children on ways to relate more creatively with their parents (Lester and Lester 1980; Ragan 1979). At another level, government-sponsored programs that provide the elderly with economic, physical, and psychological support are recommended by many social gerontologists as viable ways to reduce the middle generation's burdens, making it easier for them to satisfy their parents' needs (Butler and Lewis 1982; Cantor 1980; Cicirelli 1983; Lopata and Brehm 1981; Seelbach 1984; Shanas and Hauser 1974; Sussman 1977; Treas 1977; Treas and Bengston 1987).

Belief in the importance of maintaining strong intergenerational relations by way of government assistance is emphasized by Brody's (1980) claim that without continued public assistance, the well-being of all generations is at risk. As Treas and Bengston conclude, "Americans have come to accept that the welfare of older citizens is no longer merely a private concern, but also a public responsibility" (1987,645).

It seems to me, however, that these views have yet to distinguish between "public responsibility" and "public problem." To say that the problem is the public's responsibility means that there is something the public needs to do to help the individual while the public remains unchanged. It is another thing to say that the problem is the public's problem and something needs to be done about "the public."

Political economists of aging (critical theorists) have recognized this distinction between public responsibility and public problem and have responded, first, by rethinking the relationship between the polity, the economy, and the society (Estes, Swan, and Gerard 1984). Estes, Swan, and Gerard (1984) propose restructuring the aging policy in the United States by restructuring the class system. How will this process proceed? It will proceed by coalition building among women and men, young and old, black, brown, and white people—everyone who is a member of the disadvantaged working class in the United States.

While the interpretation of the trends presented in mainstream social gerontology provides an explanation of filial adaptation that is descriptive and possibly solvable via government assistance, it has, in my view, missed the mark. The interpretation is based on the notion that modernization has created a unique life experience for adult children. Given what has been learned about the strains in the intergenerational relationship from the qualitiative research, it is quite possible that the problem has been simplified to a general process that brushes over significant details.

In addition, a quick glance at history suggests that the mainstream's interpreation is insufficient. To begin with, the historian D.H. Fischer (1978) argues that the transition in age relations occurred in America before urbanization and industrialization, thus before modernization. The revolutionary ideals of liberty and equality, for Fischer, called into question the tradition of gerontocracy, a social system where powers and privileges are accorded by seniority; ties between generations were "snapped" as social atomism grew in the United States.

As already noted, political economists of aging have successfully placed the "aging problem" within a sociohistorical and sociopolitical context, one that defines the problem not merely in terms of "modernization" but more specifically in regard to the particular relationship between the economy and polity. Having done so, these progressive theorists have looked beyond demographics to other factors affecting the intergenerational relationship, for example, dominant values, ideologies, and the class stucture of the society (Minkler and Estes 1984).

As sketchy as the modernization idea is, it continues to dominate the subject of intergenerational relations. Even the current trend interpretation by mainstream theorists is framed around the idea of modernization which is why so much stress is placed on "public resonsibility." A more extensive review of the demographics, however, could test the accountability of the dominant interpretation.

The interpretation presupposes that (1) being old today means being dependent and therefore that more elders means more problems for contemporary adult children, especially in lieu of the family form evolving from extended to nuclear; (2) traditionally, all or most siblings shared filial responsibility; (3) before women entered the paid workforce, they had the time and energy to devote to their older parents and did so; (4) marital disruption was uncommon until recently; and (5) prior to the jet age, the United States was not a mobile society.

These presuppositions, while seemingly true to the facts, overlook important historical and cultural realities. The fact is, in most cases, that older Americans today live independent lives and are nearly as well off, if not better off, financially than their children. Although median income is less for persons sixty-five and over than for younger persons, the overall financial picture is often much better for the elderly. For instance, in 1980, 75 percent of the 17.7 million houses owned by older persons were owner occupied, most of which were owned free and clear (*Developments in Aging 1985,89*). Thanks to inflation, many adult children cannot afford the houses and other luxuries enjoyed by their parents.

If anything, senior citizens support their adult children more than the other way around. Riley and Foner (1968) found the proportion of older parents giving help to their children to exceed the proportion receiving help from them. Similarly, Hill (1970) found the older generation more likely to give money to their offspring than the reverse; six years later, Atchley (1976) found only about 3 percent of retired couples reporting cash gifts from family and friends. In a more recent study, Bankoff (1983) found that parents were the primary source of emotional support for middle-aged daughters who had been widowed.

Furthermore, the extended-to-nuclear-family argument is simply unfounded. Numerous works have dispelled the myth that the family form evolved, linearly, from the extended to the nuclear (Demos 1970; Fischer 1978; Laslett and Wall 1972; Poster 1978; Reiss 1965). In Laslett and Wall's (1972) comprehensive study of the history of the family, over 93 percent of all the households in the past, excepting in Japan, were found to consist of one or two generations, not three.

Similarly, Hareven (1987) found only 9 to 12 percent of early American urban families to be extended and that the nuclear household was not an isolated unit but one integrated with outside extended kin. Demos (1970), Greven (1970), and Smith (1979) have also established that the dominant preindustrial family structure was a modified extended one within a nuclear household. It was not uncommon for dependent elders to move into households with people other than family (Hareven 1987).

The suggestion that more siblings means more shared filial responsibility simply ignores the fact that, historically, select siblings have born the brunt of caring for frail parents. Depending on the culture and circumstance, primary caretaking has fallen upon the eldest son (and his wife) in traditional China, India, and Korea; an adult son living on the same land as his parents, which was common in colonial America; the unmarried child, the youngest child still living at home, or the child in closest proximity, as in the early history of the United States; or on daughters as, among the Italians, Jamaicans, Navaho, and early Americans (Human Area Research Files; Chudacoff and Hareven 1979; Fischer 1978; Greven 1970; Hareven 1987, 1982; Holmes 1983; Treas 1979). Even today, there is usually among siblings one, more often than not a sister, who ends up with the greater share of filial responsibility (Troll 1986).

The interpretation that before women entered the workforce they were in a better position than their contemporary counterparts to care for their parents presents a biased view of women's contributions to the family in earlier America. Ignored is the enormous task load of our grandmothers and foremothers who raised large families and managed households without current conveniences. As for child rearing, in the Plymouth Colony, married couples produced on the average eight children each.

The overall family size (free persons only) in the United States reported by the census was 5.80 in 1790; 5.28 by 1860, 4.93 in 1890, 3.77 in 1940, 3.67 in 1960, and 3.70 by 1967 (Laslett and Wall 1972). Obviously, the farther back we go in American history, the more children women bore and raised. In addition, the mean age for first marriage among women was 24 in 1650, 25 in 1800, and 23 in 1950, not a big change over the centuries (Fischer 1978). I would argue that responsibilities and role strain were no less stressful for women then than now. Surviving in preindustrial America could actually be seen as more difficult than in postindustrial America, given the lack of high technologies, medical care, and zero state support.

This is not to downplay the strains experienced by adult daughters in America today, but to place it in a historical perspective. No doubt women in this country have been the "mainstay" in supporting the aged, but the larger question would appropriately be, "Why is this so?" That is, what conditions have led to this circumstance? The correct question might be: "Are the strains daughters now experience in their relationships with their parents associated simply with caregiving and multiple role demands, or is there more to the picture than meets the eye?"

Although divorce and single parenthood were less common in days gone by, widowhood was not. To say that marital disruption is unique to today's middle-aged person is to disregard the high number of deaths among this age group in early American history. The percentage of persons in the United States surviving to age 50 from age 20 was only 58.5 percent between 1650 and 1700. By 1850, the percentage was 73.5 (Fischer 1978). Clearly, many Americans died during their early marriage-age years.

Finally, contrary to popular myth, geographic mobility is not new in the United States. The United States has always been a highly mobile society (Laslett and Wall 1972). American settlers were, after all, immigrants: people who left behind homes, families, and motherlands. The pioneers quickly moved to new frontiers, often at the cost of saying good bye to loved ones. An impressive work by Eldridge and Thomas (1964) documents the patterns of settlement in the United States and shows how, characteristically, migration has been highest among the 20–34 age group. In addition, it was an accepted practice for children to be sent to live in other households where they would work as servants or apprentices (Anderson 1971; Hareven 1982; Katz 1975). By adulthood, children were launched from their parents' households and expected to find places of their own which often meant moving into new territories (Hareven 1982).

My objection to the interpretation presented in mainstream social gerontology is not with the argument that contemporary adult children are experiencing strain in relationships with their parents, nor is it against concerns over strains emerging from caregiving to infirm parents, but with the explanations of such intergenerational strain and the accompanying expectations of individual adaptation. What has happened in mainstream literature is that the strain between generations has been defined in terms of demographics, presented as an issue of elderly dependency, and traced to modernization. Like the cause, the outcome is assumed to be an unavoidable human condition, one in which the best hope is for adult children to adapt. The problem with all of this is that, as revealed in

Part I of this book, the subject encompasses more than demographics, dependency, and modernization. Given the contribution of the interviews analyzed within a critical framework, we know there is more to the current intergenerational discord in the United States than has been presented and, thus, more to improving the outcome than has been proposed by mainstream social gerontologists.

9 MAINSTREAM
EXPLANATIONS OF
INTERGENERATIONAL
RELATIONS

The scenario in mainstream literature goes something like this:
Adult children in the United States are faced with a unique life
situation that is changing the adult child/parent relationship. The
new life situation involves unprecedented demographic, social,
economic, and cultural trends. It is not uncommon for today's adult
children to be limited in what they can do to maintain a close and
caring relationship with their parents, nor is it uncommon for them
to experience ill feelings because of this. Counseling, government
programs, and social support networks are needed to help adult
children adapt to their new life situation.

The scenario simplifies the problem, suggesting that change in
intergenerational relations is correlated with movement toward
modernity. The older American family and its problems are explained
in terms of a monolithic model. Given the "stone" character of all
that is modern, the scenario suggests that adult children, with some
governmental assistance, must reshape themselves for the sake of
intergenerational harmony. The reasoning behind this kind of analysis
originates from what I have referred to as ideological theories.

Predominant notions of the older American family are derived
from established theories of the family in sociology rooted in ideas
dating back to the nineteenth century. The common thread running
through both the legacy and the heritage is that the family is an
adapting institution that has evolved unlinearly over centuries and
that most recently has been jeopardized by rapid social change,
industrialization, and, in particular, urbanization. They are ideological theories.

The Beginnings of Ideological Theory of the Family

Influenced by Charles Darwin's work on biological evolution,
social thinkers of the nineteenth century who became known as

social Darwinists sought to explain the evolution of social forms such as the family. Social Darwinists concluded, after analyzing historical literature and to a lesser extent cross-cultural evidence of "primitive" people, that the modern family is an evolutionary form that has advanced unilinearly through different stages. Each scholar, however, determined stages differently.

In "Family Forms and Variations Historically Considered," Bardis (1964) reviews these scholars who have explored the subject of family evolution: Bachofen (1861), Maine (1861), Morgan (1877), Westermarck (1891), Spencer (1897), and Briffault (1927). Accordingly, Bachofen argued that human society began with promiscuity, progressed to gyneocracy, which was finally succeeded by a patriarchate. Maine discredited the notion of a matriarchal stage in social evolution and proposed, instead, the historical prevalence of a patriarchate. Then, Morgan divided family history into four successive stages: promiscuity, punalua, polygamy, and monogamy. Rejecting primitive promiscuity, Westermarck declared the human race as having always been monogamous. Spencer suggested that monogamy among humans is innate. Finally, Briffault claimed that primitive monogamy was the fourth stage in family evolution, the first three being group marriage, matriarchy, and patriarchy.

Bardis (1964) concludes that conclusive evidence concerning evolutionary stages does not exist, that unilinear development is fiction. One of his criticisms centers on scholars using mythology and religious writings as if they were "objective ethnological treatises." Actual fieldwork in anthropology also demonstrates that earlier constructs of unilinear evolutionism of the family are incorrect. Bardis concludes with this list of criticisms, based on ethnological studies, submitted by Margaret Mead to refute evolutionary theories: (1) Evolutionary stages are arbitrary; (2) evolutionists were biased by their own norms, thereby constituting earlier forms of family in antitheses of their own families; (3) conclusive evidence of evolutionary states is unavailable; (4) customs are functioning institutions (not mechanisms of survival of the fittest); (5) matrilineal cultures are not always less advanced; (6) combinations of family systems are common; (7) in some cultures, the status accompanying polygamy is greater than that between two spouses; and (8) it is questionable that *Homo sapiens* has instincts.

Of all the social Darwinists of the nineteenth century, Herbert Spencer was to have the greatest impact on early American sociology and its view of the family, particularly family problems. Spencer, under the influence of Auguste Comte, was a positivist, that is, he was convinced that general laws of the social order exist and that these laws can be identified by applying science, as empirical and value-free investigation, to the study of society; if determined, the social facts can yield possible solutions for social maladjustments in addition to increasing human control over nature (Horkheimer 1972; Collins and Makowsky 1972).

As a positivist, Spencer believed that the laws of evolution govern the cosmic, the biological, and the social in the same developmental totality; all evolutionism, according to Spencer, is based on the same principle. Described by Collins and Makowsky (1972), Spencer's sole principle is that "matter begins as a homogeneous mass of simple particles and gradually becomes organized as the particles come together to form heterogeneous parts of a complex whole" (1972,69). This principle suggests that all that exists evolves from the simple and unorganized to the complex and organized (Collins and Makowsky 1972). This process that changes structures cannot, wrote Spencer, "occur without changes of functions" (1897,471–489).

In applying the principle to the evolution of society—evolution being the process of environmental adaptation—Spencer explained that Western society, having evolved from preindustrial to industrial, represented the survival of the fittest. According to Spencer, the notion of adaptation through the survival of the fittest would culminate in humans and their society becoming perfected morally, intellectually, and materially. In his view, nonadaptation to environmental conditions results in evil, mental and physical misfits, and social problems that, if left to natural forces, would ultimately be destroyed. For this reason, Spencer strongly opposed any action, particularly public assistance, that would run contrary to the "laws of nature."

Similarly, Emile Durkheim (1895) proposed a positivistic method of research in which social phenomena would be systematically observed and classified as individual facts of the empirical world, having inherent properties identifiable by, yet separate from, the researcher. Strongly influenced by Spencer, Durkheim conceptualized evolution as moving from incoherent homogeneity to coherent heterogeneity, or from the simple to the complex (Coser 1977). He also agreed that a relationship existed between structures and functions. For instance, Durkheim (1921) formulated an explanation of the family by first conceptualizing the modern family as a social institution that has evolved from a simpler form; then, using cross-cultural studies, he traced the familiar institution back to its "original" form in order to answer this methodological question: What function does the family have in maintaining social order?

1900–1920: Emerging Theory of the Family in the United States

Sharing in the fervor of positivism and social evolutionism, early American sociologists were committed to exploring the natural laws ruling human behavior through reasoning and research. They assumed that social progress was the outcome of social evolution. Theirs was a moralist position in which the inescapable industrial revolution was identified as the culprit behind the perceived social problems of the time, such as women wanting rights and equality, prostitution, illegitimacy, divorce, delinquent children, child labor, and poverty. Moreover, a relationship existed between these conditions and the family (Christensen, 1964).

In 1907, William G. Sumner wrote that "the way to build a science of sociology is to build it in the same fundamental methods that have proved so powerful in the other sciences. I mean the more or less exact sciences." Relying on ethnographical data, Sumner developed his theory of social evolutionism, suggesting that customs, including monogamy and polygamy, evolve to fit particular historical situations. His study began by describing the needs of "primitive people" and extended to established ways of doing things, what he called folkways, in current day society.

Folkways, according to Sumner, are the result of trial and error in social life, tested means of societal survival accumulated over centuries; they are "the widest, most fundamental, and most important operation by which the interests of men in groups are served" (1907,43). Sumner believed that social life is largely a work of nature in which human beings adapt to their distinctive cultures,

Based on this argument, Sumner advocated a system of laissez-faire, natural liberty, and economic competition as the surest way to social progress. He opposed all forms of social programs and legislation with the exception of public education which he saw as being of "immense value . . . to society" (1907,558). Among the many social issues derided by Sumner, sexual equality was at the forefront. In primitive days, he said, women adapted themselves to men, who were physically stronger, and in so doing gained their protection; the difference between the sexes today—women responsible for the private realm, men the public—is, as then, based on necessity. Efforts to change that which has been selected by natural circumstance would, as Sumner saw it, disrupt social development.

Lester F. Ward, too, was interested in discovering the natural laws determining human behavior. But unlike Spencer and Sumner, Ward rejected the position that only natural forces play into the evolutionary process. For Ward, humans had evolved from lower forms of life, but along the way they had acquired an intellect allowing them to create a world above the natural; this higher stage of evolution acting through human consciousness is what Ward in 1883 called the "principle of social telesis." Tampering with the laws of nature to hasten progress was seen by Ward as not only acceptable but desirable.

Ward's integration of evolutionary ideas with social change led him to suggest that male sexual selection evolves from brute force to greater sensitivity with the higher location of a species on the developmental continuum. The human male, distinguishable from the animals by his cognitive development, uses foresight and reason to satisfy his female, who in turn looks to him for "that protection and those favors which he alone can confer" (1911,615). His conclusion was that the various institutions of marriage such as polygamy, polyandry, and monogamy (the best type as he saw it) unfolded in accordance with reproductive forces.

Probably the most ardent proponent of positivism among the Spencerian evolutionists in the United States was Franklin H. Giddings. He preferred using inductive procedures and quantitative methods, especially statistics, to determine the natural laws of social life. In *Principles of Sociology* (1896), Giddings presented his concept of "consciousness of kind," which referred to "a state of consciousness in which any being, whether low or high in the scale of life, recognizes another conscious being as of like mind with itself."

Consciousness of kind represented to Giddings the major principle behind human motives and the organization of society. Specifically, Giddings classified people according to the development of their consciousness of kind. On a larger scale, association produces self-consciousness and then social consciousness, which ultimately produces civilization, characterized by public and private associations. In short, consciousness of kind is the key subjective fact of social life from Gidding's viewpoint. The height of civilization occurs when the social personality is developed to such a point in its members that they, as "rational" beings, accept their social responsibilities and thus adapt to their social environment.

The foregoing heritage of family sociology was steeped in moralistic views of what constituted social problems and social progress (Collins and Makowsky 1972). Times have changed, however, and so have societal perceptions of social problems. Divorce, women's equality, and illegitimacy, for example, are socially defined as less immoral today than in the early 1900s. In fact, in some circles they are not considered problems at all and are looked on as better alternatives for individuals and society than unhappy marriages, discrimination by sex, and marriage merely for the sake of the children. But because early sociologists had their eyes on the adaptation of the individual, they could not envision either the possibility of redefining the expectations placed on the individual or radical social reform for the sake of every individual's well-being.

1920–1950: The Interactionist Perspective on the Family

That the goal of sociology is to determine scientifically the natural laws of human behavior was articulated by W.I. Thomas and Florian Znaniecki in a methodological note to their classic work, *The Polish Peasant*, first published in 1918. They believed it was possible for social scientists to discover the laws of human nature and use the obtained knowledge to control societal change for the betterment of humankind. Furthermore, they believed that the internal as well as the external workings of the family evolve. In order to go beyond a purely subjectivist or objectivist interpretation of social life, Thomas and Znaniecki focused on the interplay of individual attitudes and cultural values in order to account for family conduct. Their favored scientific approach was inductive; the case history of the family in its everyday living formed their method (Stryker 1964).

The conclusion Thomas and Znaniecki drew in *The Polish Peasant* was that family disorganization is caused when a family member's attitudes are modified from essentially "we" attitudes to "I" attitudes, that is, from having values associated with those of the family to values that are not. Once this occurs, the family cannot return to its original psychology, for what has been learned cannot be unlearned. Nevertheless, as Thomas and Znaniecki propose, "Reorganization of the family is then possible, but on an entirely new basis—that of a moral, reflective coordination and harmonization of individual attitudes for the pursuit of common purposes" (1918,1170). To summarize this solution in one word: adaptation.

Thomas wrote that the main problem of humans is "one of adjustment, and the forms of adjustive effort are 'behavior'" (1937,1). Adjustment, as he saw it, is both an individual and a group matter best understood, scientifically, as a functional and processual activity influenced by the cultural milieu. Failure to adapt is identifiable as dependency and criminal behavior in the individual and as a measure of decline in the group. In short, society requires the active adaptation of the individual which involves reasoning, imagination, and the creation of new patterns of action from the external world.

The social-psychological perspective of Thomas and Znaniecki was promoted in the work of Ernest Burgess, who in 1926 referred to the family as a "unity of interacting personalities." In other words, the family is a unit of interacting personalities tied to the community and the larger society, and its basic reality is derived from each family member's roles (Stryker 1964). For Burgess, the family develops a conception of itself in the interaction of personalities, and personalities develop via socialization, or social adaptation, which he saw as the fundamental process in the determination of social progress. From Burgess's standpoint, socialization of the person meant that the individual "consciously modifies his behavior and shapes his purposes to promote more efficient co-operative activity and to realize the higher welfare of the group," the means for making such adjustment being the role (1926,2). Socialization here has to do with the individual's roles changing in relation to new life situations. Purposeful adjustment of the individual is, as Burgess would have it, a necessary component in the social process.

There are six basic assumptions in Burgess's theory of the family. They are, as outlined by Osmond (1987): (1) Family stability is fundamental to social order; (2) family functions are in decline; (3) a duality exists between the private and public spheres; (4) marriage precedes family; (5) the family world is different from the public world; and (6) quantitative research and scientific objectivity are the appropriate methods for studying the family, hence, questionnaire surveys can accurately represent the family (i.e., family members' attitudes, values, and beliefs).

In retrospect, the interactionist theory of the family reflects the social values of the era in which it first appeared in sociology circles. Noteworthy are these objections, raised by Osmond (1987): (1) Conformity is expected at the expense of the individual; (2) social differentiation is not taken into account; (3) the contradictions of the system are ignored; (4) the interrelationship between family and society is left unaddressed, thereby maintaining the duality between the public and private realms; and (5) the survey method (as applied by interactionists) produces answers reflecting the status quo because it typically accounts for the white middle-class family in its relative stability of everyday life, having family members with zero to little experience in varied family organization or personal relationships.

Osmond explains that the interactionists regarded the work world as brutal and cold and the home world as kind and warm, a place for emotional rejuvenation. By viewing this split as natural or inevitable in advanced industrial society, family sociologists determined that a basic analysis of the interrelationship between the family and society was not the business of family theory. They did not consider important the "degree of public-private overlap among various social strata and the functionality of a public–private ideology for capitalist society" (1987,114).

From Sumner to Burgess, early American sociologists have believed in natural laws and have had "a common faith in the adaptability of the family as an institution to new social conditions" (Howard 1981,16); for them, "the family represented an adapting institution that had evolved over centuries, and the social problems were signals that family roles needed to change" (Thomas and

Wilcox 1987). These views became the tradition on which American sociologists built theories of the family.

In summary, the impact of "natural" progress on the family was at the forefront of earlier sociological subject matter. Methodologically, this was an era in which family researchers embraced wholeheartedly the scientific method, striving toward harder, systematized social facts, collecting data, for example, on women's problems, broken homes, and juvenile issues (Christensen 1964).

1950s to the Present: Structural Functionalism, Exchange Theory, and the Life-Course Perspective

Structural Functionalism

Although the interactionist, or social-psychological, framework held a prominent position in early mainstream sociology, by the second half of the twentieth century the structural functional model won out as the dominant theoretical framework of family study in the United States. The structural functional model was much inspired, though, by the notions of socialization found in the work of the interactionists. The model was also molded by the ideas of Spencer and Durkheim and their first-round followers, especially the notion about structures and functions being interdependent.

Within the model, society is regarded as a stable and well-integrated social system composed of various structures that have various functions that contribute to the equilibrium of the total organism, namely society. Under ideal conditions, all the structures are in perfect harmony with one another, each advancing the stability of the social system. If, however, there is disruption in one element (e.g., the family), then most likely other elements (e.g., the economy, religion, and the polity) will be affected, and the final result will be a shattered society. Social change from without, then, is viewed as a threat to the natural order of the society. By this model's standards, it is essential that members of a society be socialized, or taught to adapt, to societal's norms and values. Anything less would destroy the normal progression of the society.

The structural functional approach to the family, most associated with George Murdock and Talcott Parsons, regards the relationship between the family and society as a functional one. More specifically, structural functionalists view the family as a structure that performs essential functions for other institutions and, ultimately, for society. The essential functions of the family include providing food and shelter, regulating sexual behavior, replacing members, socializing children, and protecting young and old alike (Parsons and Bales 1955; and Sorokin 1966). Other functions mentioned include affection, love, and emotional support—all of which are deemed vital to human happiness and involve all members, young and old alike, in social and civil activities that help to set group boundaries (Skolnick and Skolnick 1980). Recently, Treas and Bengston (1987) wrote that "even in a fast-changing and ever more complex postindustrial society," direct caregiving, psychological support, and social contact are still important familial functions in meeting the needs of dependent elders.

Performing the necessary family functions is, of course, done by family members, who, as seen by structural functionalists, are bundles of statuses and roles. The role, as the expected behavior accompanying the status or social position, is seen as the smallest stabilizing unit of the social system. Actual role conduct of family members is guided by the individuals and their families sharing a sense of what ought to be, something that is embedded into each person's personality via socialization, a view reminiscent of the interactionist perspective. Structural functionalists take the position that family members want and need social approval, which can be secured by living up to their role expectations (i.e., conforming in such a way that family functions are satisfied).

The extent to which the family fulfills its functions is measured by its success in meeting the vital needs of the existing society. Thus the functional prerequisites of the family must occur for human society to subsist in the status quo (Reiss 1965). As Kando notes, "the family is not viewed as active in social change, but rather as a defensive survival-oriented, and adjustive entity" (1978,191). Adjustment, from this perspective, involves alteration of position and behavior (statuses and roles) in conformance with the established ways of society. Again, the responsibility for protecting society from debasement and decay is directly associated with adaptation, in this case, of family members.

Keeping the universal process of evolution always in mind and building on the ideas of their forefathers, the structural functionalists seek to understand the laws guiding everything that is society. Their search is based on the belief that phenomena, including human behavior, can be observed, classified, and described as individual facts, rather than as reciprocal parts of the totality. Based on empirical data of family life, structural functionalists have reasoned that the modern family emerged into its contemporary form, the nuclear family (which consists of wife, husband, and their dependent children), from its traditional form, the extended family (which consists of two or more generations of the same kinship living together). Most structural functionalists acknowledge the industrial revolution as the turning point between the traditional and modern family. Accordingly, the family changes dramatically as society modernizes, that is, as it is transformed from a rural way of life having limited technology, undifferentiated institutions, and a traditional outlook on life to an urban way of life having high technology, differentiated institutions and a cosmopolitan outlook emphasizing efficiency and progress (Cowgill 1974).

The modernization thesis, specifically outlined in "Aging and Modernization: A Revision of the Theory (1974)," by Donald Cowgill, proposes that in the traditional family, all social life revolves around the family unit. Family members live and work together in the same household; they educate their children, value a traditional way of life, rarely move geographically or socially, and have few elderly members to care for. Life revolves around secondary and tertiary institutions. Family members live and work in separate places and schools educate their children. They value a cosmopolitan way of life, frequently move geographically and sometimes socially, and care for many elderly members. For those who accept this argument, the modern family is an isolated unit in which members have fewer people to turn to for emotional support and elders are excluded from meaningful roles. In the opinion of Parsons and Bales (1955), the modern family is ideal for meeting the needs of industry.

In short, structural functionalists present the family as a continuous, unilinear homogeneous phenomenon and omit discussing the exact nature of society from their particular history of the industrial revolution. Their argument presupposes a specific, almost ideal-type, family structure for both traditional and modern families. It also implies that the nuclear family is the more functional family form for modern society, even though it disrupts intergenerational relations. The disruption is tolerable because it can be addressed by helping individuals help themselves; what really matters is the stability of society at large.

The tenets of structural functionalism focus on social regulation and "reflect the basic ideology of contemporary capitalist society" (Osmond 1987). For example, the theory assumes social stability is maintained through norms that reflect collective consensus. The question that these norms might mirror dominate ideology is neither asked nor answered. The theory also assumes that institutions are interrelated by their functions, which contribute to the overall working of the society. No one considers that functions and institutions might serve the interests of one group over another. Nor is there concern that roles are unaffected by power dimensions or must be fulfilled regardless of the individual's needs and desires. Instead, focus is on the question of conformity, of what is proper and expected of the individual in status quo.

Exchange Theory

In 1950, George Homans combined social evolutionism, social psychology, and structural functionalism to create his own theory of group behavior, an important theoretical development in the rise of exchange theory. The eclectic work, *The Human Group* is true to positivist tradition, separating by a "rigorous code" "concrete observation" collected from a case method into "classes of fact," which were "organically synthesized" into interrelated propositions for the purpose of developing a grandiose theory of group behavior (1950,21). Group behavior, according to Homans, consists of mutually dependent elements whose relations bring about the "seeds of emergent evolution." He studied the group, the family included, as "an organic whole, surviving and evolving in an environment" (1950,10).

Similarly, Homans's view of society was, much like Spencer's, analogous to a biological system in which groups are like organs and people like cells. In such a system there is interdependence between structure and function. In the same fashion as structural functionalists, Homans was interested in organizing elements in society (e.g., the family) in such a way that they can prosper while contributing to the "life of organized society." The question for Homans was how to have social change without social dissolution or, as Homans asked, "How can we create an adaptive society?" That is, is it possible for modern society to maintain its "complex adaptation to the natural environment" given centralized control, meaning advanced civilization (1950, 466).

To Homans, civilization is the culprit undermining primary group ties because its process redistributes activities to other institutions. The weakening of intergenerational ties, for example, was explained by Homans as resulting from the functions of the "old-fashioned family," which included extended kin, being subsumed by specific institutions, mainly the institutions of economy, education, polity, and religion, leaving the "modern urban family," which does not include extend kin, with only these functions: procreation, care of young children, and keeping a house.

Some results, Homans argues, are that fathers have lost much of their authority in the home and mothers have found their identities bound to child rearing, as it has become almost exclusively their responsibility and one of their few roles. For this reason, many women may feel overly anxious about parenting, and since the public realm has become more admired than the private, women have become dissatisfied with domestic life. Children, meanwhile, have become increasingly emotionally dependent on members of their nuclear families. These are exceptional insights into the qualitative differences in the nature of the family, even though their basis is questionable.

The continued dominance of institutions in the realm that was once the family's will, according to Homans, further family disintegration, with the consequence that children are "trained" in such a way that their adult personalities "are apt to have an impaired capacity for maintaining a steady state under stress," a condition continually perpetuated as it is passed down from one generation to the next (1950,280). Homans was convinced, however, that in gaining an understanding of group behavior through "patient analysis of the relations of mutual dependence in the internal and external systems," sociologists would work out new norms for family members, perhaps even reviving extended kin networks (1950,280).

A few years after publishing *The Human Group,* Homans advanced his ideas on human behavior in *Social Behavior: Its El-*

ementary Forms (1961); this newer work became the cornerstone of what is now known as exchange theory. As before, Homans' main interest was group behavior and interaction, only now he included the reinforcement patterns of human beings, arguing that human behavior is motivated by self-interest (i.e., individuals strive to maximize rewards and minimize costs in their interaction with others). As long as the exchange relationship is perceived as being more rewarding than taxing, the relationship continues.

Dowd (1980) expands the concept of reinforcement patterns to include the exchange of rewards and costs between younger and older generations. The problem between generations is defined by Dowd as an imbalance of power resources (e.g., money, knowledge, persuasiveness, and social position) created by the structural realities of advanced industrial society, such as retirement and the ones mentioned by Homans. In particular, Dowd suggests that the aged are at a disadvantage in modern society because, compared to the younger generation, they have fewer power resources with which to maximize their rewards. Since elders have less to offer, the younger generation views relationships with them as more costly than profitable, and for this reason, often discontinues relationships. In the end, the aged experience a high degree of social isolation and a low degree of self-esteem.

Thus, Dowd views intergenerational relations as a process of social exchange in which the older generation's social position and well-being have been undermined by circumstances accompanying twentieth-century industrial society. This theme appears many times throughout the literature on aging, especially in discussions of filial responsibility, mutual aid, and social support of the elderly. It is also a popular motif in cross-cultural studies of the aged, such as Charlotte Ikel's *Aging and Adaptation*, in which concern is with the mutual independence and reciprocity taking place within the modern family verses the traditional one. Taking after structural functionalists, proponents of exchange theory reduce the family structure to its functions, size, and hierarchy of generations, but their emphasis is on the ongoing exchange of power resources within the family and on individuals readjusting to create a more equal balance. Hence their overriding regard is with individuals adapting to their immediate environments.

In the likeness of its heritage, exchange theory captures the essence of its time. This utilitarian model amply resembles the "human capital model" so endeared as the American way (Osmond 1987). Life is the free market, the individuals the competitors, the power resources the capital. It is assumed that individuals have starting points—why they are not the same is not an issue—and end up in various social locations because of their abilities or inabilities, as the case may be, to rationalize and calculate in order to maximize personal desires. "Telling people what they already believe is a very effective way to gain a wide audience;" quotes Osmond from Mayhew (1980,352); preceding the quote, Osmond says, "It is the close fit between this individualistic social theory [exchange theory] and American ideology that makes it so imminently acceptable and obviously true" (1987,111).

Developmental or Life-Course Theory

The developmental framework is used almost exclusively today in mainstream discussions of the adult child/parent relationship. What makes this the preferred framework is that it highlights the critical periods of individual and family development and in this way accounts for change in families over time. The framework is a composite of concepts borrowed from other sociological frameworks plus these two added components: human development and historical conditions, adopted from psychology and history, respectively (Hareven 1981; Hill and Rodgers 1964; Mattessich and Hill 1987).

For example, from evolutionary theory, the developmental framework appropriates such concepts as complex whole, environmental conditions, living organisms, maladjustment, natural stages, and social evolution; from interactionism, family disorganization, family interaction, personalities, public and private domians, roles, socialization, and social process; from structural functionalism, conformity, equilibrium, institutions, norms, positions, roles, social order, stability, structure and functions, and systems; from exchange theory, costs and rewards, exchange, mutual independence, power resources, and reciprocity; from psychology, developmental stages, developmental tasks, and psychic experiences; and from history, life history analysis and sequential regularities.

These many concepts are used in the developmental framework to explain family interaction within the context of historical sequence; the favored method is the survey, with a preference for longitudinal studies. Recognized is the fact that both the individual and the family change over time; accordingly, individuals progress through developmental stages, families move through life-cycle stages, and the maneuverings affect one another—it's the evolutionists' tune with a different twist. The developmental stages noted most often are Erik Erikson's eight, which cover the entire life span and represent the individual's ability to adapt to life changes. Demographic data are primarily recalled with regard to family stages.

In discussions of the older family, Erikson's generativity, or middle-aged stage, and integrity, or older adult stage, are of concern; the primary tasks of the middle-aged person are civil responsibilities, career, and family formation, whereas finding continuity and meaning in one's life is the task of the older person. As for the family, the critical stages typically cited are marriage, birth of children, children leaving home, the postchildren period, the empty-nest phase, and the final dissolution of the marriage through the death of one spouse. Attention is on how well families cope during times of expected changes in the family's structure. All told, the stages encompass effects of maturation, circumstance, and experience, covering the entire existence of the family, and represent crucial choices for both the aging individual and the family (Neugarten 1968; Glick 1977).

Again, the adaptation theme. The developmental framework in the same manner as evolutionary theory and the theories that followed, is bound to the notion that individuals and their families must successfully adapt to conditions they encounter in this life. A quote by Hareven, a leading proponent of the life-cycle model, clearly shows that the nineteenth century torch is still burning:

> The adaptation of individuals and their families to the social and economic conditions they face when they reach old age is contingent on the paths by which they reach old age. The differences in their respective backgrounds, particularly the ways in which their earlier life

experience and their cultural heritage have shaped their
views of family relations, their expectations of support
from kind, and their ability to interact in determining
their adaptability to conditions they encounter in "old
age." (1981,143–144)

Fashioned after the interactionist perspective, the developmental framework conceptualizes the family as a unit of interacting
individuals who affect one another as well as the larger society;
personality formation, socialization, the importance of the family as
the keeper of moral order all come into play under the framework.
The carried-over ideas include believing that socially approved
behavior and expectations are learned, negotiated, and carried out
over time within the group itself; and, in the event of changing
environmental conditions, equilibrium is held to be maintained by
the discarding of old roles and the creation of new ones (Mattessich
and Hill 1987).

The central star in the family drama is the developmental task,
meaning a "task which arises at or about a certain period in the life
of an individual, successful achievement of which leads to his
happiness and to success with later tasks, while failure leads to
unhappiness in the individual, disapproval by the society, and
difficulty with later tasks" (Havighurst 1953,2). Eleanor Godfrey, a
student of Parsons, pointed out that each developmental task must
satisfy imperatives of the biological, the cultural and the personal,
thus taking the task into the realm of a functional prerequisite (Hill
and Rodgers 1964). On the one hand, family members of all ages
have their own developmental tasks, how well each task is performed
depending on how well other family members perform their tasks
(Hill and Rodgers 1964); and on the other hand, each family has its
developmental tasks (family functions), which "satisfy society's
needs for healthy, nourished societal members" (Matterssich and
Hill 1987,442).

Successful achievement of the tasks became identified with the
well-being of both the individual and society (Hill and Rodgers
1964; Havighurst 1953; Mattessich and Hill 1987). With tasks
associated with functions, developmental theorists came to regard
the family not only as an enmeshed group of interpersonal relationships but also as an institution of the larger social structure. The

dual facets of the family and accompanying adaptive features are reiterated in this remark by Mattessich and Hill: "They [families] have the capacity to adapt to changes precipitated both internally by the members themselves and externally by the larger society; and this capacity constitutes another systemic feature" (1987,441).

The structural facet of the family in the developmental framework is supported by the concepts of norms and roles. Accordingly, norms, or shared guidelines prescribing appropriate behavior in a given situation, are what link family members to society and spur developmental task accomplishments (Mattessich and Hill 1987). The idea is that changes in norms lead to changing the role content of social positions. From the developmental perspective, new historical conditions and family situations change norms, which then alter role content of positions. Another criterion is the changing age composition of the family, which is assumed to affect role expectations surrounding reciprocity among family members (Hill and Rodgers 1964).

The historical aspect of the picture is what has attracted scholars of family history to the developmental framework. The scholars have contributed to the historical dimension of the framework by examining the effects of life events and demographic circumstance on cohorts (e.g., children of the Great Depression, working-class and middle-class women of the Great Depression, and couples during World War II) and the consequence of this on the family. Impressed in their research are the realities of cultural values, economic depressions, employment practices, fertility, marriage, mortality, migration patterns, industrialization, urbanization, and wars, for example, and their direct impact on personality development, household forms, and family structures, and how these factors in turn affect family relations (Achenbaun 1978; Elder 1974; Demos 1970, 1972; Greven 1970; Hareven 1981, 1987; Laslett and Wall 1972).

Results of the work of the "developmentalists" have been helpful in disproving the myths that in the United States the nuclear family is an isolated unit and that it evolved from an extended form. Their consideration of class, ethnic, and cultural differentiations has also served to dispel family myths. But they have also served to perpetuated the idea that social forces are something humans confront, not create; this way of thinking is exemplified in Hareven's remark that historical studies of the family have "a view of people in the past as actors confronting historical forces." (1987,37).

Besides having the obvious problems of those in the other ideological theories, the developmental framework has two of its own: (1) It analyzes development of the individual without reference to how social organization shapes human personality; and (2) it focuses on historical events and circumstances as if they existed without cause (i.e., it presents history without the historical nature of society). While its proponents have established the quantitative differences in the family over time, they have missed the qualitative differences by ignoring the specific organization of society, American society, which is unlike any before it. Like other mainstream theories, developmental theory fails to make the connection between the organizational base of society and family relations. A word should be said about the countertradition in developmental theory, however, which has responded to the objections raised above, but this new tradition is not part of what has been defined in this chapter as work in the mainstream.

Limitations

The main limitation of the dominant developmental theory and other mainstream theories of the family is their positivist view of the nature of their subject matter. From evolutionary to developmental theory, a distinction has not been made between nature and second nature, between that which is biological and that which is constructed reality. Consequently, customs, events, norms, roles, institutions, social systems, developmental tasks, and all the other concepts used in the established tradition appear as empirical facts or things existing outside any human construction yet capable of being analyzed in terms of universal laws. In short, that which is social is presented as a fact of nature or as a natural and unchangeable fact of life.

This is why evolutionary theorists assume families have evolved through various stages, or why interactionists, with their subjectivist focus, view the family as the stronghold of social stability, or why structural functionalists presuppose a very specific, almost ideal-type family form for both traditional and modern families, or why exchange theorists are so comfortable portraying human interaction as "human capital," or why developmental theorists present human personality as if it were a natural phenomenon, or why all of them are preoccupied with adaptation.

Clearly, mainstream theorists make assumption after assumption about the social world based on their personal experiences and perceptions. Their theories are tools for organizing their mirrored images of the social order. Because social gerontologists' theoretical frameworks of the family are limited by their ideological underpinnings, so too are the explanations of the filial adaptation derived from them. Most definitely, if the explanations of the adult child/ parent relationship dominating mainstream social gerontology continue to be constructed from ideological theory, they will remain narrow in scope and short on inspiration.

Chapter **10**

A FINAL TESTING OF MAINSTREAM SOCIAL GERONTOLOGY

I have shown through qualitative research that the source of strain in the adult child/parent relationship goes beyond demographics to aspects of the emotional structure of the adult child/parent relationship under capitalist patriarchy. Left unanswered, however, is the extent to which baby boomers have close and caring relationships with parents according to traditional methodology. The following is a quantitative look at the adult child/parent relationship, using conventional factors for analysis.

Definitions of Terms

In the study, *baby boomers* were defined as U.S. citizens born between 1946 and 1957. *Parents* referred to the mothers and fathers of baby boomers; the category included biological parents who were not present during some or all of the baby boomer's childhood years and stepparents. *Siblings* included the sisters and brothers of the baby boomers; step-and half-sisters and brothers were included. *Filial adaptation, affectional bond, filial responsibility, filial anxiety,* and *ill feelings* were defined earlier in this work. *Intergenerational relationship* was the relationship between baby boomers and their parents.

Indicators of the "affectional bond" included sentiments of love, compassion, affection, and attachment. Expression of the bond included periodic visits, phone calls, letter writing, and shared values, in addition to protective behaviors (e.g., providing physical and financial assistance to the family member in need plus moral support). Measures of "filial responsibility" included shared living, shopping, escorting, household tasks, assistance in meeting daily needs, bureaucratic paperwork, money, and any assistance that supports a family member. Indicators of "filial anxiety" included

146

adult children feeling anxious, scared, or apprehensive in regard to their parents growing older, becoming more dependent, and dying. Finally, "ill feelings" included anger, contempt, frustration, hatred, hostility, insecurity, jealousy, resentment, and sense of burden, among others.

Sample

A nonrandom sample of fifty baby boomers was obtained through a snowball technique that proved to be very successful. Basically, I informed by word of mouth to friends, family, and members of various departments at the State University of New York at Buffalo (SUNY Buffalo) and at Alfred University of my need for volunteers. In some cases, I contacted the participant first; in other cases, it was the other way around. Many participants were helpful in giving me the names of potential participants. As it turned out, I had more people willing to give interviews than I needed. The interviews were conducted at a mutually agreed upon location; as a result, the interviews were held at a number of locations including my offices at SUNY Buffalo and at Alfred University, the participants' work places, eating establishments, my home, college classrooms, and the participants' homes. I talked with the participants before the interviews to ascertain if they indeed met the age and citizenship criteria and to brief them on the purpose of the study.

Safeguarding the confidentiality of participants was maintained throughout the study by the substitution of each participant's name with a number. During the taping of the interviews, participants were not referred to by name. The tapes, interview notes, and transcriptions were identified by number and pseudonym only. At the beginning of the interviews, the participants signed a consent form that included an explanation of how, without prejudice, they were at liberty to discontinue the interviews at any time and to refuse to answer any question they felt would make them feel uncomfortable. None did so.

Instrument

The interview was divided into a structured part and a semistructured part. In the structured part, baby boomers were asked basic demographic questions about themselves and their parents. The demographic data were acquired during the first part of the interview. The baby boomers were asked a series of open-ended questions designed to elicit whether they had close and caring relationships with their parents and why or why not this was so. These are the questions that were consistently put forward to the baby boomers:

1. Do you call your parent(s)? How often?

2. Do you write letters to your parent(s)? How often?

3. Do you visit your parent(s)? How often?

4. During your adult life, what, if any, sort of mutual aid has been exchanged between you and your parent(s)?

5. *a.* Do you feel close to your parents? Why or why not?

   b. Have you always felt close/not close to your parent(s)? Why or why not?

6. Do you share the same values as your parents? Why or why not? 7. Do you feel anxious about your parents' growing older? Why or why not?

8. *a.* Do you think of your parent(s)' mortality?

   b. If yes, does the thought of your parent(s)' mortality lead you to think of your own mortality? Why or why not?

9. Do you feel anxious about the possibility of your parent(s)' becoming more dependent? Why or why not?

10. Do you have any ill-feelings toward your parent(s)? Please explain either way.

During the first four interviews, the subject of support and approval was brought up by the participants. Thereafter, I asked the respondents these two additional questions in relation to the "ill feelings" construct: "Have your parents been supportive of you and of the things you have done throughout out life? Why or why not?" and "Do you seek your parent(s)' approval now that you are an adult? Please explain."

All interviews were taped, with the exception of six that were not taped due to the spontaneity and/or the location of the interviews (e.g., in a restaurant). All interviews were transcribed after they had been conducted; the six interviews that were not taped were transcribed immediately after they had been conducted. Local (New York State) interviews were done with me, the researcher, present. Within the state, interviews were held in Albany, Alfred, Andover, Buffalo, and Rochester. Other interviews were conducted in Connecticut, Kansas, and Oregon.

The interviews from Connecticut and Oregon essentially followed a format in which participants, without a researcher present, went down the list of questions and answered them into a tape recorder. Interestingly, the participants from Connecticut and Oregon were, in general, more willing to discuss their familial relationships in depth, especially with regard to aspects they considered unpleasant. I attribute this to the social expectation that adult children are supposed to have good relations with their parents, and thus people are inhibited about expressing ill feelings toward their parents to a stranger. The interviews from Kansas were conducted while I was there on business. The interviews extended over an eight-month period.

The responses were categorized into four relation categories: affection, filial responsibility, filial anxiety, and ill feelings. Responses to affection were categorized as no contact/some+ contact; don't feel close/feel somewhat+ close, don't share values/share some+ values, no support/some+ support. Responses to filial responsibility were categorized as no mutual aid/some+ mutual aid; filial anxiety categories included no anxiety to parent(s) growing older/some+ anxiety to parent(s) growing older, no anxiety to parent(s)'s mortality/some+ anxiety to parent(s)' mortality, and no anxiety to parents becoming more dependent/some+ anxiety to parents becoming more dependent. Finally, responses to ill feelings were categorized as no ill feelings/some+ ill feelings. Frequency counts were taken of the categories and then described.

In order to analyze the traditional notion of "adaptation" among the baby boomers, the categories adapted/nonadapted were devised. "Adapted" characterized baby boomers who, in regard to their parents, felt close, were responsible, did not experience filial anxiety, and did not have any ill feelings. The "nonadapted" category was for the baby boomers who answered in the negative to one or more of the relation categories.

The Quantitative Findings

Profile of Sample

The sample population was more heuristic than anticipated in that it included individuals from an array of backgrounds in terms of educational levels, geographic locations, occupations, marital arrangements, and family arrangements. Of the 50 baby boomers interviewed, 33 were female and 17 were male; 42 were white of which 5 had Jewish backgrounds; 1 was black, 1 was part-Asian, 1 was part-Spanish, another was part-Native American, black, and white, and 4 were part-Native American. The educational levels of the baby boomers ranged from high school to graduate/professional school, as shown in Table 1.

Table 1
Educational Levels of the Baby Boomers

Educational Level	*N*
High school	1
Some college	7
Technical/vocational	5
Two-year college	3
Four-year college	19
Graduate/professional school	15

As for where the baby boomers grew up, the baby boomers were scattered throughout the United States although nearly half came from New York State. Table 2 shows this diversity.

Table 2
States Where Baby Boomers Grew Up

State	*N*	State	*N*
Alabama	1	New York	24
California	3	No. Carolina	1
Connecticut	2	Oklahoma	2
Illinois	1	Ohio	2
Kansas	2	Oregon	2
Massachusettes	1	Tennessee	1
Minnesota	1	Texas	1
Montana	1	Virginia	1
Missouri	1	Washington	1
NewMexico	1	Wisconsin	1

At the time of the interviews, 2 of the baby boomers were living in an urban area in Connecticut, 1 in rural Kansas, 31 in rural New York, 8 in urban New York, and 8 in Oregon; their occupational categories ran the gamut; see Table 3.

Table 3
Occupation of Baby Boomers

Occupation	N
Mechanic/technician/welder/carpenter	6
Artists	10
Homemakers	5
College professors	4
School teachers	2
Clerical	5
Owned or worked in business	4
Nursing/medical technician	6
Librarian	2
Editor	1
Clergy	1
Student	1
Town clerk	1
Therapist	1
Herbalist	1

The years the baby boomers were born included years from 1946 to 1957. Table 4 presents this distinction.

Table 4
Birthdates of Baby Boomers

Year of Birth	N	Year of Birth	N
1946	4	1952	6
1947	4	1953	4
1948	1	1954	6
1949	9	1955	5
1950	4	1956	2
1951	3	1957	2

Regarding the marital status of the baby boomers, there was a fair mix of statuses (see Table 5). Of the married population, 17 had spouses who were employed full-time; 26 of the baby boomers had children. Two were single parents.

Table 5
Marital Status of Baby Boomers

Marital Status	N
Married	25
Remarried/1 Divorce	4
Divorced	1
Single/Never Married	15
Single/1 Divorce	3
Single/2 Divorces	1
Separated	1

Most of the baby boomers had siblings, though 5 did not; of the baby boomers who had siblings, 27 had a least one sibling living near their parents. The breakdown of the number of siblings is shown in Table 6.

Table 6
Sibling Status of Baby Boomers

Sibling Status	N
No sibling	5
One sibling	7
Two siblings	16
Three siblings	11
Four or more siblings	11

Furthermore, of the 50 baby boomers, 17 lived near their parents; of these, 2 daughters had their mothers living with them and 1 son was living with his parents, and 35 had parents who were both still living, 12 had only their mothers, and 2 only their fathers, 13 also had mothers and 11 had fathers who were in poor health, and 22 had both parents living who were both in good health.

Only 11 of the 50 baby boomers had at least one parent still employed full-time in the paid labor force. The residence of the baby boomers' parents extended across the United States (see Table 7). Table 7 totals to only 48 because being that one baby boomer's mother was living in New York and her father in Vermont, and another baby boomer had parents buried in New York.

Table 7
State Residence of Baby Boomers' Parents

Parents' State	N	Parents' State	N
California	3	New York	20
Connecticut	2	Ohio	2
District of		Oklahoma	2
Columbia	1	Oregon	1
Florida	3	South Carolina	1
Kansas	2	Tennessee	1
Massachusettes	1	Texas	1
Minnesota	1	Vermont	1
Missouri	1	Washington	1
New Hampshire	1	Wisconsin	2
New Mexico	1		

A total of 29 baby boomers during their childhood years had mothers who were full-time homemakers, 3 had mothers who worked part-time outside the home, the rest had mothers who were employed full-time in the paid labor market. Occupations of fathers are accounted for in Table 8.

Contact

In Tables 9 to 20, answers to questions on the extent to which baby boomers have close and caring relationships with their parents are presented, beginning with frequency of contact and ending with extent of ill feelings.

Table 8
Occupation of Baby Boomers' Fathers

Father's Occupation	N	Father's Occupation	N
Engineer	6	Draftsman	2
Executive/owned		Pilot	1
Business	5	Graphics designer	1
Factory worker	8	Postal carrier	1
Salesman	4	College professor	4
Own small		Lawyer	2
business	2	Writer	1
Journalist	1	Middle-management	3
Rancher	2	Grocer/clergy	1
Minister	1	Psychiatrist	1
Ship navigator	1	Dentist	1
Not mentioned	2		

Table 9
Percentage of Visits with Parents

Frequency	%	Frequency	%
Daily	8	Once every 6 months	4
Several times a week	4	Once a year	14
Once a week	14	Once every 2 years	8
Once every 2 weeks	2	Once every 3 years	4
Once a month	8	Weekly during summer	4
Once every 2 months	6	Varies	6
Once every 3 months	10	Not reported	2
Once every 4 months	6		

All the baby boomers maintained some contact with their parents. As you can in Table 9, the majority (76 percent) of the baby boomers visited their parents at least once a year, and almost a quarter of them visited their parents at least once a month. Frequency of contact was affected by geographic distance, as revealed in the interviews. All the baby boomers who visited their parents not more than once every two years lived in different states from their parents, whereas those who saw their parents on a weekly basis lived in the same community as their parents.

Table 10
Percentage of Letter Writing to Parents

Frequency	%
None	62
Once a week	6
Once every 2 weeks	2
Once a month	6
Once every 2 months	4
Once every 6 months	2
Varies	18

Letter writing was the least-favored medium for intergenerational contact, as indicated in Table 10. As many as 62 percent of the baby boomers did not engage in letter writing with their parents. Only 14 percent wrote to their parents at least once a month. Given that 66 percent of the baby boomers reported that they did not live in the

Table 11
Percentages of Phone Calls with Parents

Frequency	%
Daily	4
Lives With Parents	6
Three times a week	8
Twice a week	10
Once a week	34
Once every 2 weeks	12
Once a month	14
Once every 2 months	2
Once every 3 months	2
Once every 4 months	2
Varies	6

same area as their parents, letter writing frequency is low. But, phone calls more than made up the slack. Nearly 90 percent of the baby boomers said that they talked to their parents over the phone at least once a month, and 60 percent of them reported talking to their parents at least once a week (see Table 11).

Assistance

In many families, the baby boomers did not need to assist their parents because their parents were capable of managing for themselves one way or another; some parents hired outside assistance for tasks related to household management, health care, and mental health, for example, and many parents received financial assistance through public and private old age assistance programs. Still, as can be seen in Table 12, a full 88 percent of the baby boomers reported that they provided some assistance for their parents, of which only 8 percent gave financial support.

The tasks provided varied with each participant; a few examples cited in the interviews included mowing the lawn, visiting a sick parent in the hospital, painting the house, watching pets while parents go on vacation, providing moral support during emotionally difficult times, running errands, and doing the laundry.

Table 12
Percentage of Baby Boomers Providing Assistance to Parents

Assistance Reported	%
Miscellaneous[a]	80
Miscellaneous & Financial	8
None	12

[a]Miscellaneous includes any one of a multitude of tasks aside from financial support provided by the baby boomers to help their parents (e.g., yard work, house maintenance, emotional support, and errands).

In terms of financial support, the baby boomers were definitely more on the receiving than the providing end: 68 percent of the baby boomers cited situations in which their parents had assisted them financially as adults, for example, providing downpayments for a house or car, buying furniture, helping with college loans, and paying for moving expenses (see Table 13). Other parental support reported by the baby boomers included baby sitting, house sitting, pet sitting, and running errands, to name a few.

Table 13
Percentage of Baby Boomers Receiving Assistance
from their Parents

Assistance Reported	%
Miscellaneous[a]	20
Miscellaneous & Financial	68
None	12

[a]Miscellaneous includes anyone of a multitude of tasks outside of financial support provided by the parents to help the baby boomers, e.g. baby sitting, emotional support, errands, and house sitting.

Close to Parents

It is clear from the data in Table 14 that more of the baby boomers felt closer to their mothers (80 percent) than to their fathers (60 percent), a difference of 20 percent. Interestingly, only 4 percent of the baby boomers said that they did not feel close to their mothers, compared to 32 percent who said the same about their fathers. The percentage of baby boomers who said they felt close to their mothers today though there was a time when they did not, was 8 versus only 4 percent expressing this sentiment toward their fathers. But the percentages for the close but not close/neutral category were higher for the mothers (8 percent) than for the fathers (4 percent).

Values

The typical response of the baby boomers, 68 percent, was that they shared some but not all the values of their parents, as exhibited in

158   AGING PARENTS, AMBIVALENT BABY BOOMERS

Table 14
Percentage of Baby Boomers Close to Parents

Closeness	%
Close to mother	80
Close to mother now (not always)	8
Close and not close to mother/neutral	8
Not close to mother	4
Close to father	60
Close to father now	4
Close and not close to father/neutral	4
Not close to father	32

Table 15. Common values shared included fairness, honesty, and loyalty; as one baby boomer remarked, "the common decency stuff." Where the differences lie were in values about sexual behavior, environmental issues, racism, and sexism, about which the baby boomers regarded themselves as being more liberal than their parents. Only 22 percent of the baby boomers said that they shared the same values as their parents without any qualifications. Left were 10 percent of the sample who said that they flat out did not share the same values as their parents.

Table 15
Percentage of Baby Boomers Sharing Same Values as Their Parents

Share Values	%
Yes	22
Some/Basically	68
No	10

Anxious about Parents

The baby boomers were basically divided on the question of whether they felt anxious about their parents' growing older: 54 percent said yes and 46 percent said no (see Table 16). Of the 54 percent who answered in the affirmative, however, only 6 percent spoke of the anxiety in terms of being overwhelmed with the responsibility of caretaking; the other 48 percent mentioned other reasons for their concern, such as not wanting to see their parents suffer, not wanting their parents to become vulnerable, not wanting one of their parents to outlive the other, and thereby leave the survivor alone and lonely, and not wanting to lose a parent. Thus, if the "compassion" factor is taken into account in the anxiety response, then in actuality only 6 percent of the baby boomers suffered from "filial anxiety."

Table 16
Percentage of Baby Boomers Anxious about Parents' Growing Older

Anxiety	%
Yes	54
No	46

Anxious About Mortality

Table 17 shows that the baby boomers are thinking about their own mortality, 78 percent of them in this study. But under 25 percent of the baby boomers said that they thought of their own mortality in relation to thinking about their parents' growing old and dying. Many other reasons were given for what led the baby boomers to think about their own mortality; for instance, 7 women told me that they became anxious about their own mortality after giving birth to their first child, 1 man related his awareness of mortality to his stint in the Peace Corps, 1 woman said she became interested in death and dying during an Indian vision, and another related her consciousness of death to her husband's recent stay in the hospital. Again, the profile of the sample does not support the notion of filial anxiety among the baby boomers.

Anxious about Parents' Dependency

The data in Table 18 suggest that the baby boomers are anxious about their parents' becoming more dependent; the percentage of the

Table 17
Percentage of Baby Boomers Thinking about Own Mortality

Thinking of Own Mortality	%
Yes	78
No	22
In relation to Parents' Mortality	%
Yes	24
No	76

baby boomers who felt anxious in this regard was 40. Thus 60 percent did not report feeling anxious about the possibility of their parents' becoming more dependent with age. And again, of the population answering yes, most were more concerned about their parents' well-being than they were about the likelihood of personal strains accompanying caretaking.

Table 18
Percentage of Baby Boomers Anxious about
Parents Becoming Dependent

Anxious	%
Yes	40
No	60

Ill Feelings

Well over half (56 percent) the baby boomers declared having some ill feelings toward their parents, and an additional 18 percent explained that at one time they had ill feelings toward their parents, but for one reason or another they had overcome them. As divulged in Table 19, only 26 percent of baby boomers alleged that they had never experienced any ill feelings toward their parents. Worth noting is that of the 74 percent of the baby boomers who mentioned having some ill-feelings toward their parents, either currently or in the past, 52 percent gave follow-up statements qualifying the actions of their parents that had created the ill feelings.

Table 19
Percentage of Baby Boomers Having Ill Feelings
Toward Parents

Ill Feelings	%
Yes	56
Not now	18
No	26

Adapted Adult Children

Baby boomers who maintained contact with their parents felt close to both their mothers and fathers, shared the same values as their parents, did not feel anxious about their parents' growing older or becoming more dependent, or about mortality, and never experienced any ill feelings toward their parents were classified, according to the traditional notion of filial adaptation, as "adapted adult children." There were 8 (16 percent) of them in this study, 7 males and 1 female, meaning that 41 percent of the males versus 3 percent of the females in this study fit the perfect adaptation category. A profile of these 8 baby boomers shows both similarities and differences between them:

> Five of the eight baby boomers lived in different states fromtheir parents (though one lived in the same area as his parent during the summer months), whereas one of the other three lived with his parents and the other two lived in the same community as their parents; all of them were residing in rural communities in upstate New York. Seven were white; one was white and Native American; three had completed technical school; three had B.A. degrees, and two had earned their M.F.A.s.; all eight were employed full-time; their occupations were kiln technician, machine shop technician, welder, glass sculptor/professor, librarian assistant, carpenter, pro-

duction ceramists, and potter, respectively; five were married and three were single; of the five who were married, two had marital partners who were employed outside the home; two had widowed fathers, one had a widowed mother who had remarried, and the other five had parents who were still alive and married to each other; only four claimed to have both a mother and a father in good health; all had siblings except for one (number of siblings per baby boomer was eight, four, two, zero, two, two, three, and three, and the number of siblings living near the parents was one, four, one, zero, two, two, zero, and two, respectively); and all had parents who were retired from full-time paid employment outside the home.

Nonadapted Adult Children

The other 42 baby boomers (84 percent) in this study fell short in one or more of the traditional adaptation constructs and thus were classified as "nonadapted adult children." Nevertheless, none of the baby boomers fits the perfectly unadapted category, that is, adult children who do not maintain contact with their parents, do not feel close to both mothers and fathers, do not share the same values as parents, feel anxious about parents' growing older or becoming more dependent, or about mortality, and who experience ill feelings toward parents. In looking at the sample population profile in general, it is clear that the remaining population is a diverse group of individuals who are not perfectly adapted for a mixture of reasons.

It is apparent that there are strains in the intergenerational relationship under investigation. It is also obvious that something other than demographics is behind the strain in the intergenerational relationship; otherwise, the "adapted" baby boomers would neatly fit the demographic expectations spelled out in mainstream social gerontology, specifically surrounding the number of siblings, women being in the paid labor force, marital arrangements, and geographic mobility. In fact, the "adapted" children in this study included an individual who had as many as eight brothers and sisters and another who had none, individuals who had spouses employed outside the home and individuals who did not, and an individual who lived with his parents and others who lived in states far away from their parents. On the other side, some "nonadapted" adult children fit the demographic expectations while others did not. Moreover, the variation (20 percent) in the closeness claimed toward mothers and fathers could not be accounted for with demographics. Also curious is the contrast between closeness and ill feelings. A majority of the baby boomers said that they felt close to their mothers (80 percent) and fathers (60 percent), while a majority also admitted to having ill feelings now or within their adult lifetime toward their parents (74 percent). It would appear from this study that it is typical for adult children simultaneously to experience closeness and a degree of ill feelings toward their parents.

Of course, the reason for the discrepancy has to do with the special character of the adult child/parent relationship under capitalist patriarchy, which creates ambivalent feelings in the adult child. The reason we understand the ambivalence is not because of the quantitative research but because of the qualitative content of the interviews having been analyzed from a critical framework.

In this book I have shown the importance of examining the adult child/parent relationship qualitatively within a critical framework. It is clear that the emotional structure of the intergenerational relationship is incomprehensible using the mainstream approach, which ignores the social organization of society. The ambivalence experienced by the baby boomers is a product of capitalist patriarchy, and it is indicative of strain in the adult child/parent relationship. If my research had been confined to the mainstream model, this would never have been understood. Without insight into the emotional structure of the intergenerational relationship from a critical perspective, proposed solutions to strain between the generations will continue to be inadequate. For this reason, I am critical of the mainstream approach and its accompanying filial adaptation.

My position is that the notion of filial adaptation reflects an ideology regarding human nature. Filial adaptation is a problem, but a problem not of the individual, as insinuated in mainstream gerontology; rather, it is a political problem stemming from the current social organization of American society. Filial adaptation warns us that something is amiss in our society. I believe that an evaluation of the adult child/parent relationship that accounts for the emotional structure of the family under capitalist patriarchy is necessary for understanding strains in the adult child/parent relationship in the United States today. Ambivalence in adult children is a reality we need to address, and to do so we cannot ignore capitalist patriarchy.

BIBLIOGRAPHY

Achenbaum, A. 1978. *Old Age in the New Land.* Baltimore: Johns Hopkins University Press.

Adams, B. 1968. *Kinship in an Urban Setting.* Chicago: Markham.

Adorno, T. 1973. *Negative Dialectics.* New York: Seabury.

Adorno. T., E. Frenkel-Brunswik, D. Levinson, and R. Sandford. 1969. *Authoritarian Personality.* New York: Norton.

Agger, B. 1976. On happiness and the damaged life. In J. O'Neill, ed., *On Critical Theory.* New York: Seabury.

————. 1979. *Western Marxism and Introduction: Classic and Contemporary Sources.* Santa Monica: Goodyear.

Albrecht, R. 1954. Relationships of older parents and their children. *Marriage and Family Living* 16:33–37.

Anderson, M. 1971. *Family Structure in Nineteenth-Century Lancashire.* Cambridge: Cambridge University Press.

Anetzberqer, G. 1987. *The Etiology of Elder Abuse by Adult Offspring.* Springfield, Ill.: Charles C Thomas.

Arato, A., and E. Gebhardt, eds. 1987. *The Essential Frankfurt School Reader.* New York: Continuum.

Atchley, R. 1976. Orientations toward the job and retirement adjustment among women. In J.F. Gubrium, ed., *Time,Roles, and Self in Old Age.* New York: Behavioral Publications.

————. 1976. *The Sociology of Retirement.* Cambridge, Mass.: Schenkman.

Bankoff, E. 1983. Aged parents and their widowed daughters: a support relationship. *The Gerontologist* 38:226–230.

Bardis, P. 1964. Family forms and variations historically considered. In H. Christensen, ed., *Handbook of Marriage and the Family.* Chicago: Rand McNally.

Barrett, M. 1980. *Women's Oppression Today: Problems in Marxist Feminist Analysis.* London: Verson.

Bengston, V. 1979. Research perspectives on intergenerational interaction. In P.K. Ragan, ed., *Aging Parents.* Los Angeles: University of California Press.

Bengston, V., and N. Cutler. 1976. Generations and intergenerational relations: perspectives on age groups and social change. In V. Bengtson and E. Shanas, eds., *Handbook of Aging and the Social Sciences.* New York: Van Nostrand Reinhold.

Bengston, V., and J. Dowd. 1980. Sociological functionalism, exchange theory and life cycle analysis. *International Journal of Aging and Human Development* 12(1):55–73.

Bengston, V., and A. Kuypers. 1971. Generational differences and the developmental stake. *Aging and Human Development* 2:246–260.

Bengston, V., and R. Manuel. 1976. *Ethnicity and Family Patterns in Mature Adults: Effects of Race, Age, SES and Sex.* Paper presented at the annual meetings of the Pacific Sociological Association, San Diego.

Bengston, V., and S. Schrader. 1981. Parent-child relations. In D. Mangen and W. Peterson, eds., *Handbook of Research Instruments in Social Gerontology*, vol. 2. Minneapolis: University of Minnesota Press.

Benston, M. 1969. The political economy of women's liberation. *Monthly Review* 21(4).

Benton, J. 1981. *The New Sensibility.* University of California at Los Angeles. Unpublished ms.

Blau, Z. 1973. *Old Age in a Changing Society.* New York: New Viewpoints.

Blenkner, M. 1965. Social work and family relationships in later life with some thoughts on filial maturity. In E. Shanas and G. Streib, eds., *Social Structure and the Family.* Englewood Cliffs, N.J.: Prentice-Hall.

Boszormenyi-Nagy, I., G. and Spark. 1973. *Invisible Loyalties: Reciprocity in Intergenerational Therapy.* New York: Harper and Row.

Bowlby, J. 1979. *The Making and Breaking of Affectional Bonds.* New York: Tavistock.

Bristol, L. 1915. *Social Adaptation.* Cambridge, Mass.: Harvard University Press.

Brody, E. 1966. The aging family. *The Gerontologist* 6:201–206.

———. 1980. *New directions in health and social supports for the aging.* Paper presented at the annual meetings of the Anglo-American Conference, Fordham University, New York.

———. 1981. "Women in the middle" and family help to older people. *The Gerontologist* 21(5):471–479.

Brody, E., and C. Schoonover. 1986. Patterns of parent-care when adult children work and when they do not. *The Gerontologist* 26:372–381.

Brooks-Gunn, J., and B. Kirsh. 1984. Boundaries of midlife. In G. Baruch and J. Brooks-Gunn, eds. *Women in Midlife.* New York: Plenum Press.

Browne, C., and R. Onzuka-Anderson. 1985. *Our Aging Parents: A Practical Guide to Eldercare.* Honolulu: University of Hawaii Press.

Brubaker, T., and E. Brubaker. 1981. Adult child and elderly parent household: issues in stress for theory and practice. *Alternative Lifestyles* 4:242–256.

Burgess, E. 1916. *The Function of Socialization in Social Evolution.* Chicago: University of Chicago Press.

———. 1926. The family as a unit of interacting personalities. *Family* 7:3–9.

Butler, R., and M. Lewis. 1982. *Aging and Mental Health.* 3rd ed. St. Louis: Mosby.

Cantor, M. 1975. Life space and the social support system of the inner city elderly of New York. *The Gerontologist* 15:23–27.

———. 1980. *Caring for the frail elderly: impact on family, friends, and neighbors.* Paper presented at the annual meeting of the Gerontological Society of America.

Carlsson, G., and K. Karlsson. 1970. Age cohorts and the generation of generations. *American Sociological Review* 35:710–718.

Chodorow, N. 1978. *The Reproduction of Mothering: Psychoanalysis and the Sociology of Gender.* Berkeley: University of California Press.

Christensen, H. 1964. Development of the family field of study. In H. Christensen. ed., *Handbook of Marriage and the Family*. Chicago: Rand McNally.

Chudacoff, H., and T. Hareven. 1979. From the empty nest to family dissolution. *Journal of Family History* 4 Spring: 59–63.

Cicirelli, V. 1981. *Helping Elderly Parents: Role of Adult Children*. Boston: Auburn House.

————. 1983. Adult children and their elderly parents. In T. Brubaker, ed., *Family Relationships in Later Life*. Beverly Hills, Calif.: Sage.

————. 1986. A comparison of helping behavior to elderly parents of adult children with intact and disrupted marriages. In L. Troll, ed., *Family Issues in Current Gerontology*. New York: Springer.

Cohen, S., and B. Gans, B. 1978. *The Other Generation Gap: The Middle-Aged and Their Aging Parents*. Chicago: Follett.

Collins, R. 1975. *Conflict Sociology: Toward an Explanatory Science*. New York: Academic Press.

Collins, R., and M. Makowsky. 1972. *The Discovery of Society*. New York: Random House.

Cowgill, D. 1974. Aging and modernization: a revision of the theory. In J. Gubrium, ed., *Late Life*. Springfield, Ill.: Charles C Thomas.

Cowgill, D., and L. Holmes, eds. 1972. *Aging and Modernization*. New York: Appleton-Century-Crofts.

Coser, R., ed. 1974. *The Family: Its Structures and Functions*. 2nd ed. New York: St. Martin's Press.

Coser, L. 1977. *Masters of Sociological Thought*. 2nd ed. New York: Harcourt Brace Jovanovich.

Dalla Costa, M., and S. James, S. 1972. *The Power of Women and the Subversion of the Community*. Bristol, England: Falling Wall Press.

Demos, J. 1970. *A Little Commonwealth: Family Life in Plymouth Colony*. New York: Oxford University Press.

————. 1972. Demography and psychology in the historical study of family-life: a personal report. In P. Laslett, ed., *Household and Family in Past Time*. Cambridge: Cambridge University Press.

Deutscher, I. 1968. The quality of postparental life. In B. Neugarten, ed., *Middle age and Aging*. Chicago: University of Chicago Press.

————. 1987. Misers and wastrels: perceptions of the Depression and yuppie generations. Presented paper (SA).

Donovan, J. 1986. *Feminist Theory: The Intellectual Traditions of American Feminism*. New York: Ungar.

Dowd, J. 1975. Aging as exchange: a preface to theory. *Journal of Gerontology* 15:303–27.

————. 1980. *Stratification Among the Aged*. Monterey, Calif.: Brooks/Cole.

Durkheim, E. 1895/1964. *The Rules of Sociological Method*. New York: Free Press.

————. 1921/1965. A Durkheim fragment: the conjugal family. Trans. G. Simpson. *American Journal of Sociology* 5:527–536.

Duvall, E. 1957. *Family Development*. Philadelphia: Lippincott.

Ehrlich, C. 1981. The unhappy marriage of marxism and feminism: can it be saved? In L. Sargent, ed., *Women and Revolution: A Discussion of the Unhappy Marriage of Marxism and Feminism*. Boston: South End Press.

Elder, G., Jr. 1974. *Children of the Great Depression: Social Change in Life Experience*. Chicago: University of Chicago Press.

————. 1975. Age differentiation and the life course. *Annual Review of Sociology* 1:165–190.

Eldridge, H., and D. Thomas. 1964. *Population Redistribution and Economic Growth, United States, 1870–1950*. Vol. 3. Philadelphia: American Philosophical Society.

Elshtain, J. 1981. *Public Man, Private Woman*. Princeton: Princeton University Press.

Engels, F. 1884/1972. *The Origin of the Family, Private Property and the State*. In R. Tucker, ed., *The Marx-Engels Reader*. New York: Norton.

Erikson, E. 1950. *Childhood and Society*. New York: Norton.

————. 1968. Generativity and ego integrity. In B. Neugarten, ed., *Middle Age and Aging*. Chicago: University of Chicago Press.

Estes, C., and R. Newcomer. 1983. *Fiscal Austerity and Aging: Shifting Government Responsibility for the Elderly*. Beverly Hills, Calif.: Sage.

Estes, C., J. Swan, and L. Gerard. 1984. Dominant and competing paradigms in gerontology: towards apolitical economy of aging. In M. Minkler and C. Estes, eds., *Readings in the Political Economy of Aging*. Farmingdale, New York: Baywood.

Fengler, A., and V. Wood. 1972. The generation gap: an analysis of studies on contemporary issues. *The Gerontologist* 12:124–28.

Fischer, D. 1978. *Growing Old In America*. New York: Oxford University Press.

Fraser, N. 1987. What's critical about critical theory? The case of Habermas and gender. In S. Benhabib and D. Cornell, eds. *Feminism as Critique on the Politics of Gender*. Minneapolis: University of Minnesota Press.

Freud, S. 1965. *A General Introduction to Psychoanalysis*. Trans. J. Riviere. New York: Washington Square Press.

Fromm, E. 1932/1987. The method and function of analytic social psychology. In A. Arato and E. Gebhardt, eds., *The Essential Frankfurt School Reader*. New York: Continuum.

Giddings, F. 1896. *Principles of Sociology*. New York: Macmillan.

Gilligan, C. 1982. *In a Different Voice: Psychological Theory and Women's Development*. Cambridge, Mass.: Harvard University Press.

Glick, P. 1977. Updating the life cycle of the family. *Journal of Marriage and Family* 39:5–13.

Gottlieb, B. 1981. *Social Support Strategies: Guidelines for Mental Health Practice*. Beverly Hills, Calif.: Sage.

————. 1983. *Social Support Strategies: Guidelines for Mental Health Practice*. Beverly Hills, Calif.: Sage.

Gramsci, A. 1971. *Selections from the Prison Notebooks*. New York: International Publishers.

————. 1972. *The Modern Prince and Other Writings*. New York: International Publishers.

Gray, E. 1982. *Patriarchy as a Conceptual Trap*. Wellesley, Mass.: Roundtable Press.

Greven, P. 1970. *Four Generations: Population, Land, and Family in Colonial Andover, Massachusetts*. Ithaca: Cornell University Press.

Grollman, E., and S. Grollman. 1978. *Caring for your Aged Parents*. Boston: Beacon Press.

Halpern, J. 1987. *Helping Your Aging Parents: A Practical Guide for Adult Children*. New York: McGraw-Hill.

Hareven, T. 1977. Family time, historical time. *Daedalus* 106(Spring):57–70.

———. 1981. Historical changes in the timing of family transitions: their impact on generational relations. In R. Fogel, E. Hatfield, S. Kiesler, and E. Shanas, eds. *Aging: Stability and Change in the Family*. New York: Academic Press.

———. 1982. *Family Time and Industrial Time*. New York: Cambridge University Press.

———. 1987. Historical analysis of the family. In M. Sussman and S. Steinmetz, eds., *Handbook of Marriage and the Family*. New York: Plenum Press.

Harris, L. and Associates. 1975. *The Myth and Reality of Aging in America*. Washington, D.C.: National Council on Aging.

Hartmann, H. 1981. The unhappy marriage of Marxism and feminism. In L. Sargent, ed., *Women and Revolution: A Discussion of the Unhappy Marriage of Marxism and Feminism*. Boston: South End Press.

Hartsock, N. 1981. Staying alive. The Quest Staff, ed., *Building Feminist Theory: Essays from Quest, a Feminist Quarterly*. New York: Longman.

———. 1983. *Money, Sex, and Power: Toward a Feminist Historical Materialism*. New York: Longman.

Havighurst, R. 1953. *Human Development and Education*. New York: Longman.

Held, D. 1980. The changing structure of the family and the individual: critical theory and psychoanalysis. In *Introduction to Critical Theory: Horkheimer to Habermas*. Berkeley: University of California Press.

Hess, B., and J. Waring. 1978. Changing patterns of aging and family bonds in later life. *Family Coordinator* 27(4):303–314.

Hill, R. 1970. *The Strengths of Black Families*. New York: Emerson Hall.

Hill, R., N. Foote, J. Aldous, R. Carlson, and R MacDonald. 1970. *Family Development in Three Generations*. Cambridge, Mass.: Schenkman.

Hill, R., and R. Rodgers. 1964. The Development Approach. In H. Christensen, ed., *Handbook of Marriage and the Family*. Chicago: Rand McNally.

Hogan, D. 1881. *Transitions and Social Change*. New York: Academic Press.

Holmes, L. 1983. *Other Cultures, Elder Years: An Introduction to Cultural Gerontology*. Minneapolis, Minnesota: Burgess.

Homans, G. 1950. *The Human Group*. New York: Harcourt, Brace.

———. 1961. *Social Behavior: Its Elementary Forms*. New York: Harcourt Brace.

Hooker, S. 1976. *Caring for Elderly People: Understanding and Practical Help*. London: Routledge and Kegan Paul.

Horkheimer, M. 1964. On the concept of freedom. *Diogenes* 53:73–81.

———. 1972. *Critical Theory*. New York: Herder and Herder.

————. 1980. Studies on authority and family. In D. Held, *Introduction to Critical Theory*. Berkeley: University of California Press.

Horkheimer, M., and T. Adorno. 1972. *Dialectic of Enlightenment*. New York: Herder and Herder.

Howard, R. 1981. *A Social History of American Family Sociology, 1865–1940*. Conn.: Greenwood Press.

Ikels, C. 1983. *Aging and Adaptation: Chinese in Hong Kong and the United States*. Hamden, Conn.: Shoe String Press.

Jacoby, R. 1975. *Social Amnesia*. Boston: Beacon Press.

Jaggar, A. 1983. *Feminist Politics and Human Nature*. Totowa, N.J.: Rowman and Allenheld.

Johnson, E., and B. Bursk. 1977. Relationship between the elderly and their adult children. *The Gerontologist* 17:90–96.

Jones, L. 1980. *Great Expectations: America and the Baby Boom Generation*. New York: Coward, McCann, and Georghegan.

Kalish, R. 1969. The young and old as generation gap allies. *The Gerontologist* 9:69–89.

Katz, M. 1975. *The People of Hamilton, Canada West: Family and Class in a Mid-Nineteenth-Century City*. Cambridge, Mass.: Harvard University Press.

Kando, T. 1978. *Sexual Behavior and Family Life in Transition*. New York: Elsevier.

Korbin, F. 1976. The fall of household size and the rise of the primary individual in the United States. *Demography* 13:127–138.

Lachman, M. 1984. Methods for a life-span developmental approach to women in the middle years. In G. Baruch and J. Brooks-Gunn, eds., *Women in Midlife*. New York: Plenun Press.

LaRocco, J., J. House, and J. French, Jr. 1980. Social support, occupational stress and health. *Journal of Health and Social Behavior* 21:202–218.

Lasch, C. 1977. *Haven in a Heartless World: The Family Besieged*. New York: Basic Books.

Laslett, P., and R. Wall, eds. 1972. *Household and Family in Past Time*. Cambridge, Mass.: Cambridge University Press.

Lester, A., and J. Lester. 1980. *Understanding Aging Parents*. Philadelphia: Westminister Press.

Linzer, N. 1986. The obligations of adult children to aged parents: a view from Jewish tradition. *Journal of Aging and Judaism* 1(1):34–48.

Lopata, H. 1970. The social involvement of American widows. *American Behavioral Scientist* 14:41–48.

————. 1973. *Widowhood in an American City*. Cambridge, Mass.: Schenkman.

————. 1979. *Women as Widows: Support Systems*. New York: Elsevier.

Lopata, H., and H. Brehm. 1981. *Widowhood: From Social Problem to Federal Program*. New York: Praeger.

Lukacs, G. 1968. *History and Class Consciousness*. Trans. R. Livingstone. Cambridge, Mass.: MIT Press.

Mancini, J., and R. Blieszner. 1989. Aging parents and adult children: research themes in intergenerational relations. *Journal of Marriage and the Family* 51:291–301.

Mannheim, K. 1952. The problem of generations. In D. Kecskeneti, ed., *Essays in the Sociology of Knowledge*. London: Routledge and Kegan Paul.

Marcuse, H. 1955. *Eros and Civilization*. New York: Vintage.

————. 1964. *One-Dimensional Man*. Boston: Beacon.

————. 1968. *Negations*. Boston: Beacon Press.

————. 1969. *Counterrevolution and Revolt*. Boston: Beacon.

————. 1970. *Five Lectures*. Boston: Beacon Press.

————. 1972. *An Essay on Liberation*. Harmondsworth, England: Penguin.

Marshall, V. 1983. Generations, age groups, and cohorts: conceptual distinctions. *Canadian Journal of Aging* 2(2):109–120.

Marx, K. 1974. *The Grundrisse: Foundations of the Critique of Political Economy*. New York: Random House.

Marx, K., and F. Engels. 1848/1932. *Manifesto of the Communist Party*. New York: International Publishers.

Mattessich, P., and R. Hill. 1987. Life cycle and family development. In M. Sussman and S. Steinmetz, eds., *Handbook of Marriage and the Family*. New York: Plenum Press.

Mayhew, B. 1980. Structuralism versus individualism, part I: shadowboxing in the dark. *Social Forces* 59:335–375.

Minkler, M. 1984. Introduction. In M. Minkler and C. Estes, eds., *Readings in the Political Economy of Aging*. New York: Baywood.

Minkler, M., and C. Estes. 1984. *Readings in the Political Economy of Aging*. New York: Baywood.

Moss, S. 1983–1984. The impact of parental death on middle aged children. *Omega* 14(1):65–75.

Mutran, E., and D. Reitzes. 1984. Intergenerational support activities and well-being among the elderly: a convergence of exchange and symbolic interaction perspective. *American Sociological Review* 49(1):117–130.

Myles, J. 1984. *Old Age in the Welfare State: The Political Economy of Public Pensions*. Boston: Little, Brown.

Neugarten, B. 1968. *Middle Age and Aging: A Reader in Social Psychology*. Chicago: University of Chicago Press.

Nicholson, L. 1987. Feminism and Marx integrating kinship with the economic. In S. Benhabib and D. Cornell, eds., *Feminism as Critique: On the Politics of Gender*. Minneapolis: University of Minnesota Press.

Osmond, M. 1987. Radical-critical theories. In M. Sussman and S. Steinmetz, eds., *Handbook of Marriage and the Family*. New York: Plenum Press.

Otten, J., and F. Shelley. 1976. *When Your Parents Grow Old: Information and Resources to Help the Adult Son or Daughter Cope with the Problems of Aging Parents*. New York: Funk and Wagnalls.

Palmer, R., and J. Colton. 1971. *A History of the Modern World*. 4th ed. New York: Knopf.

Palmore. E. 1978. When can age, period and cohort be separated? *Social Forces* 57(1):282–295.

Parsons, T., and R. Bales. 1955. *Family, Socialization and Interaction Process*. Glenco, Ill.: Free Press.

Pearline, L., E. Menaghan, M. Lieberman, and J Mullan. 1981. The stress process. *Journal of Health and Social Behavior*.

172   AGING PARENTS, AMBIVALENT BABY BOOMERS

Pifer, A., and L. Bronte. 1986. *Our Aging Society*. New York: Norton.

Piven, F., and R. Cloward. 1982. *The New Class War*. New York: Pantheon.

Poster, M. 1978. *Critical Theory of the Family*. New York: Seabury.

Quinn, W. 1984. Autonomy, interdependence, and developmental delay in older generations of the family. In W. Quinn and G. Hughston, eds., *Independent Aging: Family and Social Systems Perspective*. Rockville, MD.: Aspen.

Ragan, P., ed. 1979. *Aging Parents*. Los Angeles: University of California Press.

Reich, W. 1949. *Character Analysis*. 3rd ed. New York.

———. 1933/1975. *The Mass Psychology of Fascism*. Trans. V. Carfagno. Harmondsworth, England: Pelican.

———. 1980. *Character Analysis*. In D. Held, *Introduction To Critical Theory*. Berkeley: University of California Press.

Reiss, I. 1965. The universality of the family: a conceptual analysis. *Journal of Marriage and the Family* November, 443–452.

Riley, M., and A. Foner. 1968. *Aging and Society*. Vol 1. New York: Russell Sage Foundation.

Ritzer, G. 1983. *Sociological Theory*. New York: Alfred A. Knopf.

Robinson, B., and M. Thurnher. 1979. Taking care of aged parents: a family cycle transition. *The Gerontologist* 19:586–593.

Rosow, I. 1967. *Social Integration of the Aged*. New York: Basic Books.

Ryder, N. 1965. The cohort as a concept in the study of social change. *American Sociological Review* 30(6):834–861.

Seelbach, W. 1977. Gender differences in expectations for filial responsibility. *The Gerontologist* 17:421–25.

———. 1978. Correlates of aged parent's filial responsibility expectations and realizations. *The Family Coordinator* 27(4):341–350.

———. 1984. Filial responsibility and the care of aging family members. In W. Quinn and G. Hughston, eds., *Independent Aging: Family and Social Systems Perspective*. Rockville, Md.: Aspen.

Seelbach, W., and W. Sauer. 1977. Filial responsibility expectations and morale among aged parents. *The Gerontologist* 17(6):492–499.

Shanas, E. 1973. Family-kin networks and aging in cross-cultural perspective. *Journal of Marriage and the Family* 35:505–511.

———. 1977. *National Survey of the Aged: 1975*. Chicago: University of Illinois.

———. 1979. Social myth as a hypothesis: the case of the family relations of old people. *The Gerontologist* 19(1):3–9.

———. 1980. Older people and their families: the new pioneers. *Journal of Marriage and the Family* 42:9–15.

Shanas, E., and G. Streib, G., eds. 1965. *Social Structure and the Family: Generational Relations*. Englewood Cliffs, N.J.: Prentice-Hall.

Shanas, E., and P. Hauser. 1974. Zero population growth and the family of older people. *Journal of Social Issues* 30:79–92.

Silverstone, B. and A. Burack-Weiss. 1983. *Social Work Practice with the Frail Elderly and Their Families: The Auxiliary Function*. Springfield, Ill.: Charles C Thomas.

Silverstone, B., and H. Hyman. 1976. *You and Your Aging Parent*. New York: Pantheon.

Simos, B. 1975. Adult children and their aging parents. *Social Work* 18:78–85.

Skolnick, A., and J. Skolnick. 1980. *Family in Transition.* 3rd ed. Berkeley: Little, Brown.

Smith, D. 1979. Life course, norms and the family system of older Americans in 1900. *Journal of Family History* 4:285–298.

Sorokin, P. 1966. *Sociological Theories of Today.* New York: Harper and Row.

Spencer, H. 1884. *The Principles of Sociology.* New York: Appleton-Century-Crofts.

————. 1897. *The Principles of Sociology.* Abridged. Vol. 1. New York: Appleton-Century-Crofts.

Spitzer, A. 1973. The historical problem of generations. *American Historical Review* 78:1353–1385.

Spradley, J. 1980. *Participant Observation.* New York: Holt, Rinehart and Winston.

Steinmetz, S. 1978. The politics of aging, battered parents. *Society,* July-August, 54–55.

————. 1981. Elder abuse. *Aging* 315/316: 23–26.

Steinmetz. S., and O. Amsden. 1983. Dependent elders, family stress, and abuse. In T. Brubaker, ed., *Family Relationships in Later Life.* Beverly Hills, Calif.: Sage.

Stoller, E. 1983. Parental caregiving by adult children. *Journal of Marriage and the Family* 45(4):851–858.

Streib, G. 1965. Intergenerational relations: perspectives of the two generations on the older parent. *Journal of Marriage and the Family* 27:469–476.

Streib, G., and R. Beck. 1980. Older families: a decade review. *Journal of Marriage and the Family* (November):937–939.

Stryker, S. 1964. The interactional and situational approaches. In H. Christensen, ed., *Handbook of Marriage and the Family.* Chicago: Rand McNally.

Stueve, A., and L. O'Donnell. 1984. The daughters of aging parents. In G. Baruch and J. Brooks-Gunn, eds., *Women in Midlife.* New York: Plenum Press.

Sumner, G. 1907. *American Journal of Sociology.* VOL. 12. (March):598.

————. 1961. *Folkways.* New York: Mentor.

Sussman, M. 1965. Relationships of adult children with their parents in the United States. In E. Shanas and G. Streib, eds., *Social Structure and the Family: Generational Relations.* Englewood Cliffs, N.J.: Princeton-Hall.

————. 1976. The family life of old people. In R. Binstock and E. Shanas, eds., *Handbook of Aging and the Social Sciences.* New York: Van Nostrand Reinhold.

————. 1977. Family, bureaucracy, and the elderly individual: an organizational/linkage perspective. In E. Shanas and M. Sussman , eds., *Family, Bureaucracy and the Elderly.* Durham, N.C.: Duke University Press.

Sussman, M., and L. Burchinal. 1968. Kin family network: unheralded structures in current conceptualizations of family functioning. In B. Neugarten, ed., *Middle Age and Aging.* Chicago: University of Chicago Press.

Thomas, D., and J. Wilcox. 1987. The rise of family theory. In M. Sussman and S. Steinmetz, eds., *Handbook of Marriage and the Family.* New York: Plenum Press.

Thomas, W. 1937. *Primitive Culture.* New York: McGraw-Hill.

Thomas, W., and F. Znaniecki. 1918. *The Polish Peasant in Europe and America.* Chicago: University of Chicago Press.

Tong, R. 1989. *Feminist Thought: A Comprehensive Introduction.* Boulder, Colo.: Westview Press.

Townsend, P. 1968. The emergence of the four-generation family in industrial society. In B. Neugarten, ed., *Middle Age and Aging.* Chicago: University of Chicago Press.

Treas, J. 1977. Family support systems for the aged. *The Gerontologist* 6:486–491.

————. 1979. Socialist organization and economic development in China: latent consequences for the aged. *The Gerontologist* 19:34–43.

Treas, J., and V. Bengtson. 1987. The family in later years. In M. Sussman and S. Steinmetz, eds., *Handbook of Marriage and the Family.* New York: Plenum Press.

Troll, L. 1971. The family of later life. *Journal of Marriage and Family* 33:263–90.

————, ed. 1986. *Family Issues in Current Gerontology.* New York: Springer Pub.

Troll, L., and J. Smith. 1976. Attachment through the life span: some questions about dyadic bonds among adults. *Human Development* 19:156–170.

Troll, L., S. Miller, and R. Atchley. 1979. *Families in Later Life.* Belmont, Calif.: Wadsworth.

Turner, R. 1976. The real self: from institution to impulse. *American Journal of Sociology* 81:989–1016.

Ward, L. 1911. *Dynamic Sociology.* Vol 1. New York: Appleton.

Woehrer, C. 1982. The influence of ethnic families on intergenerational relationships and later life transitions. *Annals of the American Academy of Political and Social Science* 464:65–78.

Wynne, E. 1986. Will the young support the old? *Society* 23(6):41–47.

ABOUT THE AUTHOR

Jayne E. Maugans completed her Ph.D. in sociology at the State University of New York at Buffalo in 1990. She holds a bachelor's degree and master's degree in sociology from Wichita State University. As a graduate student, she directed the 11th Annual Governor's Conference on Aging in Kansas. Her master's thesis was among the first in the discipline to explore the social construction of the so called Social Security crisis. For the past four years, she has been teaching sociology in New York at Alfred University and Houghton College, specializing in gerontology, gender, stratification, and as of late, developmental studies. Recently Dr, Maugans has been appointed Associate Professor of Sociology and Coordinator of the Sociology Program at Houghton College. Along with teaching sociology and directing a learning center, she has several works in progress, one of which is on legality and the aged. Her perspective remains critical. She and her husband, Bob Scherzer, live in the country with their many animals.

INDEX

177